# FRACTURE-PROOF YOUR BONES

## A COMPREHENSIVE GUIDE TO OSTEOPOROSIS

**JOHN NEUSTADT, ND**

Published by:
LiveFullOut Media, LLC
San Diego, CA

A portion of the profits of every book sold supports charities that empower the health and education of women and children.

ISBN: 978-0-578-35696-9

Library of Congress Control Number: 2022909258

I dedicate this book to all my patients, blog readers, podcast listeners and family members who've entrusted me to help them fight the scary diagnoses of osteopenia and osteoporosis. Thank you for teaching me, inspiring me and giving me one of my most important professional missions.

# Contents

# Bones, Really?

Before going to medical school, I worked as a journalist in Chile and San Francisco. I love learning, and journalism gave me the opportunity to explore and write about topics that captured my curiosity. I thought that I wanted to be an investigative journalist covering environmental issues. But the more I wrote, the more I realized that without a background in science I would never understand the data and I'd be more susceptible to manipulation by my sources. I had an overwhelming desire to be able to fact check what I was being told and reading in the scientific research. My Literature degree didn't prepare me for that.

In 1993 I enrolled in a postbaccalaureate science program at the University of Washington where I spent another three years getting a BS in Botany. I focused on the molecular and cellular biology of plants and on ethnobotany, which is the study of how societies use plants in commerce, in manufacturing and for food and medicine.

While going through the program, two things happened. First, I realized I didn't want the life of a journalist anymore. Second, I fell in love with science and the study of using natural products in medicine. I took my premed courses during that time and eventually enrolled in naturopathic medical school because it provided the most rigorous integrative medical education I could find.

Among the dozens of doctors who trained me, two made the biggest impact. It wasn't their technical knowledge, although they were both exceptional clinicians. It was their understanding of what it took to be exceptional.

The late Thomas Dorman, MD owned Paracelsus Clinic in Federal Way, Washington. He was known as one of the fathers of Prolotherapy, a medical procedure for musculoskeletal pain. With physical exam and patient skills honed over more than four decades of clinical practice, he was also a brilliant general practice doc.

Often at the end of the day I'd patiently sit across from him at his desk as he charted. Lost in my own thoughts, I'd wait for him to talk to me. One day he stopped charting and looked at me and said, "It's always OK to say to a patient, I don't know. But then it's your duty to find out and let them know."

I have no idea what inspired him to share that with me, and I'll never know. Several years after I graduated, Dr. Dorman died. Nearly 20 years later, those words still guide me.

William (Bill) Mitchell, ND was a co-founder of my medical school, Bastyr University. He was my instructor for Advanced Therapeutics, a required class in our final year. It was an opportunity to review cases and discuss potential therapeutic options—lifestyle changes, diet, exercise, botanicals, pharmaceuticals, surgery, labs, imaging and referrals to specialists.

He'd also answer students' general questions about clinical medicine and building a practice. One day someone asked about whether they should specialize. He answered, "You won't choose your patients. They'll find you. They'll choose you. And if you listen well enough, they'll tell you what they need."

Every day I spent with those doctors was a Master Class.

When I opened my private practice in Bozeman, Montana in late 2005, my schedule started filling up with chronically sick patients who had been struggling with their health for years. They tried everything conventional medicine had to offer, yet they were still sick. Some had been to the Mayo Clinic, the Cleveland Clinic and other top hospitals around the country.

Patients came in with irritable bowel syndrome (IBS), depression, attention deficit hyperactivity disorder (ADHD), recurring infections, osteoarthritis, Lupus, Ulcerative Colitis (UC) and Crohn's disease. Within a couple of years, I'd earned the reputation as "The Doctor of Desperation". Through word of mouth, patients were finding me. I can't tell you the number of times patients told me I was their last hope. After spending years and far too much money on medicine that didn't work, they were looking for a different and scientifically rigorous way to approach their health. Doctors started reaching out to me for consults and referring their toughest cases. I loved the challenge and the satisfaction that came with helping patients have health breakthroughs.

Then my osteoporotic mother-in-law fell and broke her femur, despite taking the medication Fosamax for years. Like most patients, when she reviewed her improving bone density test results with her doctor, she was excited. My mother-in-law was convinced she had the best possible care for her osteoporosis. She didn't. But at the time, I didn't know it. And neither did she or her doctor.

Then another patient with osteoporosis came in. And another, and another. I asked them—and the thousands of patients since then—about the treatment plans their doctors provided. What I heard shocked me. There was no discussion of diet. They were told they should exercise, but not provided any resources on how to do so safely or effectively. There was rarely an evaluation of the other medications they were taking and whether they could be contributing to their osteoporosis.

Occasionally a patient would say they were told that hand-rails in their bathrooms could help prevent them from falling and breaking a bone. But they weren't told about the other dangers in their homes that the National Academy of Obstetricians and Gynecologists warns about. There was also no counseling about dietary supplements beyond simply taking calcium and vitamin D.

To do the best possible job for my patients, I started digging into the research on fracture risk and osteoporosis. The more I read, the clearer it became. The focus was all wrong.

My patients, doctors and the public had been advised to focus on bone density. But bone density is just a number on a test. The most dangerous effect of osteoporosis is breaking a bone, and the bone density test does not do a great job of predicting fractures. It's simply not

> The more I read, the clearer it became. The focus was all wrong.

as helpful as people think. I review this research in Chapter 1.

It became clear to me that the entire clinical focus needed to be on reducing fracture risk. That wasn't happening then and it's still not happening today. I hope this book helps change that.

## Down the Rabbit Hole

One of my favorite books is Lewis Carroll's *Alice's Adventure in Wonderland*. First published in 1865, it's never gone out of print and has been translated into 97 languages. It's the tale of a girl named Alice who, feeling bored and drowsy while sitting on the riverbank with her older sister, follows a talking rabbit down a hole. Thus starts the fantastical adventure where she encounters new characters. Some are helpful, some aren't and she's not sure where she's being led and where it will all end.

That's what research is like for me. It's a fun and addictive adventure of discovery as I search the more than 20 million studies catalogued in the National Library of Medicine (NLM) PubMed database. I'll read a paper, move onto the studies cited in it, and then the research cited by the next studies, and so on. What I discovered with osteoporosis is that conventional medicine's unbelievably narrow approach to treating the disease is leaving tens of millions of people dangerously uneducated and woefully unprotected.

> Conventional medicine's unbelievably narrow approach to treating osteoporosis is leaving tens of millions of people dangerously uneducated and woefully unprotected.

More than 15 years after first heading down that rabbit hole, I've become an expert in osteoporosis, written professional and consumer articles on the topic, taught physicians at medical conferences, been interviewed on podcasts and am a member of the Bone Health & Osteoporosis Foundation Corporate Advisory Roundtable.

I hadn't planned on any of that when I was in medical school. I also hadn't planned to start a dietary supplement company. But as I searched for ways to help my patients, I learned about the power of MK4, a nutrient that maintains bone strength. Since there wasn't a product on the market that provided the effective dose shown in clinical trials to work, I created it.

I started NBI (nbihealth.com) in 2006, and Osteo-K launched a year later, along with other products my patients needed. Osteo-K provides 45 mg of MK4 plus calcium and vitamin D3. Since then, Osteo-K has become one of the most recommended dietary supplements for bone health used by integrative clinicians and has shipped to people in more than 15 countries around the world. I review the research on MK4 and other nutrients in Chapter 11.

For those of you looking for a blueprint to improve your bone health, to learn how to advocate for yourself with your healthcare provider and to reduce your fracture risk, I wrote *Fracture-Proof Your Bones: A Comprehensive Guide to Osteoporosis* for you. This book is divided into two parts. In the first six chapters, I help you understand osteoporosis, your risks for fractures and how to work with your healthcare providers to get the care you need and deserve. In the second half, I share practical steps you can take as part of a comprehensive approach to growing stronger bones and reducing fracture risk.

Think of this book as your Osteoporosis Master Class. I've devoted the lion's share of my career to finding out how bones work, which conventional and integrative approaches are most effective and how you can reduce your fracture risk. And now I'm giving all I've learned to you.

But everyone knows that scientists are always making new discoveries. Make sure to sign up for my newsletter at nbihealth.com to get the latest research and health tips directly into your inbox.

To your health!

Dr. John Neustadt, ND

## Chapter 1

# What Medicine Got Horribly Wrong

Osteoporosis was first defined as a disease of low bone mineral density (BMD) in 1940 by Fuller Albright, MD, of Massachusetts General Hospital. Women are at highest risk for osteoporosis after menopause when their ovaries stop producing estrogen. When Dr. Albright simulated menopause in pigeons by removing their ovaries, he observed that their bone mass decreased, which he called "too little bone in bone."[1] How can something we've known about since the 1940s have such terrible statistics? How have we failed so miserably?

The answer is simple: Doctors have been, and still are, treating the numbers on a test and not the patient sitting in front of them. Most doctors focus solely on treating a patient's BMD test result. But in doing so, they're leaving patients dangerously unprotected.

> Doctors have been, and still are, treating the number on a test and not the patient sitting in front of them.

## BMD and Fracture Risk

A BMD test is done using a technology called dual x-ray

absorptiometry (DEXA). The DEXA scan is the gold standard for osteoporosis screening and diagnosis. When you get one of these tests, you'll see your T- and Z-scores. A T-score compares your bone density to a healthy 20–29-year-old (when bone mass is at its peak) of the same gender and race.

So if you're a 62-year-old woman, your T-score is how your bone density compares to a 20-something woman of the same race. In contrast, a Z-score compares a patient's BMD to the average bone density of someone of your same age bracket and sex.

While a Z-score can tell you if you have bone loss compared to someone your own age, a T-score is used to diagnose osteoporosis. This has been the case since 1994 when the World Health Organization defined osteoporosis as a T-score of -2.5 and osteopenia as a T-score of -1 to -2.5.[2] Although the DEXA test provides accurate and precise measures of BMD at specific sites, including the lumbar spine (L1-4), proximal femur (upper leg and hip) and forearm, the results are only as useful as they are predictive of the most dangerous thing about osteoporosis—breaking a bone.

Each year more than 300,000 Americans over 65 years old are hospitalized for hip fractures; of those, three-quarters are women.[3] The consequences are deadly. If you have osteoporosis and break a hip there's up to a 36% chance that you'll be dead within a year, and your risk for dying is increased for the next ten years.[4,5]

Even if you're one of the lucky ones who survives, your difficulties are just beginning. There's a 60% chance you'll never get back to your pre-fracture level of mobility and will require long-term care. One year after a hip fracture, 27% of patients who survive still need assistance to move around, like using a walker, cane or wheelchair.[6] Debilitating pain in the elderly is often attributed to fractures from osteoporosis and can lead to further disability and an early death.[7,8]

Therefore, *every* thought and discussion about osteoporosis—whether it's ordering a test, recommending a treatment or helping empower someone to take steps to improve their odds—must focus on reducing fracture risk. Not doing so is malpractice, or rather it should be.

> Every thought and discussion about osteoporosis—whether it's ordering a test, recommending a treatment or helping empower someone to take steps to improve their odds—must focus on reducing fracture risk.

## The Most Important Question

Doctors are talking almost exclusively to patients about how to increase their bone density. But they're missing the elephant in the room, and most patients don't understand enough to ask the most important question: "How well does a DEXA scan predict fractures?"

The short answer is, not very well. This isn't new information. We've known since 1996 that bone density predicts less than half of patients who will break a bone.[9] A 2008 study reviewed all of the previous studies on this subject and con-

**Bone density tests only predict 44% of women and 21% of men who will break a bone.**

cluded that bone density tests only predict 44% of women and 21% of men who will break a bone.[10] In fact, organizations like the North American Menopause Society (NAMS) that have published position statements on the issue have concluded that fracture risk depends on factors largely other than bone density.[11]

I'm not against bone density tests. Despite its limitations, the test results are an important piece of the puzzle. People at risk for osteoporosis, or who have already been diagnosed, should get them. The problem is not with the test. The problem is that doctors focus almost exclusively on improving bone density while excluding more important fracture risks like a patient's balance, strength and making sure they're not taking medications that cause osteoporosis and fractures.

To improve the ability to predict fractures, researchers in the 1990s began working on a model that could simultaneously analyze multiple risk factors and provide a probability of breaking a bone within 10 years. They initially struggled to get funding for this project, but eventually grants from Alliance for Better Bone Health, GE Lunar, Hologic, Pfizer, Roche, Novartis, the International Osteoporosis Foundation and the International Society for Clinical Densitometry made it possible for them to continue their work.

They had to answer a lot of questions to create their model and figure out the math to predict fracture risk using multiple independent variables. Some of the questions included: How important is smoking? Is having other diagnoses important? If so, which ones? What if someone is taking other medications? Are certain medications more dangerous than others? Their undertaking was massive. It took epidemiologists, clinicians, mathematicians, statisticians and economists 18 years to create a free, online tool, called FRAX®.

Launched in April 2008, FRAX now performs about six million calculations for people in 173 different countries each year.[12] A running tally on the FRAX website shows that since June, 2011 the FRAX calculator has assessed 35,972,572 people.

FRAX is based on patient models and evaluates your age, height and weight, femoral neck BMD, whether you've had a prior osteoporotic fracture, if one of your parents had an osteoporotic fracture, if you currently smoke tobacco, if you've ever had long-term glucocorticoid (eg, prednisone, dexamethasone) therapy, if you have rheumatoid arthritis (RA) and if you have three or more alcoholic drinks per day. Since risk factors can vary based on your country and race, calculators exist for specific regions and countries.

Creating FRAX was an impressive accomplishment, but how accurate is it at predicting osteoporotic fractures? Turns out, pretty darn good. When researchers looked at data from nearly 20,000 men and women (ages 70-90 years old) in Norway, they found that those with the lowest FRAX risk score (<4% probability of having a fracture within 10 years) were much less likely to break their hip compared to those with the highest FRAX risk score (>12% probability of having a fracture within 10 years).[13] Additional studies have also confirmed its ability to predict fractures. However, as you'll learn in this book, other medications and risk factors not considered in a FRAX risk assessment are also important.

You can calculate your 10-year risk at https://www.sheffield.ac.uk/FRAX. Since fracture risk can change based on where you live, make sure to select your region and country from the Calculation Tool drop-down menu at the top.

I've had countless conversations with scared patients who had been seeing other doctors for their osteoporosis. Despite the massive amount of evidence supporting an integrative approach, every one of them said the same thing: their doctor only talked to them about their bone density and their only advice was to take a pharmaceutical. Several patients even told me that their doctors threatened to stop working with them if they didn't take the drug. If exercise was mentioned, it typically was only as a passing comment. As you'll read in subsequent chapters, however, exercise can actually increase your risk for fractures if not done right. And while pharmaceutical interventions may be appropriate, there's so much more people can do to grow stronger bones and reduce their fracture risk. After nearly two decades of research and clinical experience, I believe the best approach is based on understanding your unique risk factors and approaching the disease holistically.

> After nearly two decades of research and clinical experience, I believe the best approach is based on understanding your unique risk factors and approaching the disease holistically.

## Why You Shouldn't Rely Solely on Your Physician

Primary care providers are the healthcare practitioners who most commonly screen eligible patients for osteoporosis. Unfortunately, when it comes to osteoporosis, these medical providers are failing. To be fair to these well-intentioned and incredibly hard-working men and women, they want to do right by their patients. Yet their limited education and the restrictions placed on them by insurance companies keep them from doing their best work.

Many doctors simply don't feel confident having in-depth discussions about anything other than drug therapies. Conversations around the commonly understood benefits of exercise and diet are complicated and time-consuming. Most doctors don't have the education to have those talks with confidence and ease and the economics of healthcare discourages it.

While the situation is slowly changing with value-based care—where insurance companies are transitioning to reimburse based on outcomes—healthcare providers who take insurance are still primarily compensated on volume, not outcomes. Since the outcome for osteoporosis treatment is increasing BMD instead of doing everything we can to decrease fracture risk, the financial incentives are skewed in an unhealthy way.

In a primary care practice, the bottom line is volume. The more patients a doctor sees in an hour, the more income they make. A 2019 survey of physicians in Sweden showed that confusion about osteoporosis, not feeling confident about how to talk about more holistic approaches and the pressure to see lots of patients in a day contributed to the inadequate treatment of osteoporosis.[14] I don't believe the situation in the U.S. is any different.

Regardless of the reason, the healthcare system is failing to address this problem. One study that looked at trends in patient bone density testing over several years estimated that 70% of eligible women and 94% of eligible men aren't getting screened for osteoporosis with a bone density scan.[15] For older patients on Medicare, the situation is even worse. Studies have concluded that 94.5% of the eligible Medicare population aren't getting bone density scans.[16-18]

To make the situation even more difficult and dangerous, osteoporosis is a silent disease. There aren't any outward symptoms that your bones are slowly getting weaker until one day, SNAP! You break a bone. When a patient who is 50 years or older breaks a bone, especially if it's a postmenopausal woman or someone on certain medications or with medical conditions that weaken bones, a doctor should screen them for osteoporosis with a bone density scan. Sadly, that's not happening. Even in patients most at risk for osteoporosis (over 65 years old), 83% of women and 96% of men don't get screened for the disease even when they break a bone.[19]

> Osteoporosis is a silent disease. There aren't any outward symptoms that your bones are slowly getting weaker until one day, SNAP! You break a bone.

Conventional medicine is falling short in another, incredibly dangerous way.

Doctors are unwittingly creating osteoporosis and fractures with the medications they're prescribing for other conditions. Many medications directly and indirectly damage bone. Prescription and over-the-counter drugs can also impair muscle strength and balance. This makes it more likely that people taking them will fall. Ninety-five percent of fractures are caused by falls, so putting patients—especially elderly patients—on medications that increase their chance of falling is a recipe for disaster.[20] Shockingly, a 2021 study funded by the National Institutes of Health (NIH) found that 94% of older adults (65 years and older) are prescribed medications that do just that.[21]

**Doctors are unwittingly creating osteoporosis and fractures with the medications they're prescribing for other conditions.**

In Chapter 4, I review your risk factors for osteoporosis and fractures, and in Chapter 5 I take a deep dive into medications that weaken bones and cause them to break. But before we get there, let's look a bit closer at the problem of osteoporosis in the U.S. and globally.

## Chapter 2

# A Global Health Crisis

Osteoporosis is the most common bone disease in the world, affecting more than 200 million people, including 53 million in the U.S.[1,2] It's so common that every 30 seconds someone in the world with osteoporosis breaks a bone.[3] Your risk for osteoporosis and fractures increase the older you get, and we're all getting older. Since the global population is aging, the number of people with this dangerous disease is rapidly increasing. To put the situation into a bit more of a global perspective, let's look at osteoporosis in a few regions around the world.

> Osteoporosis is so common that every 30 seconds someone in the world with osteoporosis breaks a bone.

## United States of America

Osteoporosis mostly affects postmenopausal women, but men can still get it. In the U.S., more than half of women 50 years old and up and 41% of men 65 years or older have significant bone loss.[4] While it's a tremendous problem now, it's nothing compared to what's coming. We're on the cusp of a tsunami of new cases and the personal and national devastation they'll create.

From 2010-2019 in the United States alone, the 65-and-older population grew by more than a third, and by 2050 there will be an estimated 84 million Americans in that age group.[5,6] This trend isn't isolated to the U.S. It's happening in every country. By 2050 the number of people around the world 65 years and older will grow by nearly 480%, from 323 million to 1.55 billion.[7]

Osteoporosis is second only to cardiovascular disease as a global problem.[8] In the U.S., osteoporosis creates more disability than high blood pressure, breast cancer, rheumatoid arthritis, stomach cancer, pancreatic cancer, ovarian cancer and Parkinson's disease.[9]

> In the U.S., osteoporosis creates more disability than high blood pressure, breast cancer, rheumatoid arthritis, stomach cancer, pancreatic cancer, ovarian cancer and Parkinson's disease.

If you're a woman, your risk for breaking a bone because of osteoporosis is equal to your combined risk for breast, uterine and ovarian cancer.[10] And if you're 50 years old or older, your risk of dying from a hip fracture is similar to your risk of dying from breast cancer.[8] Osteoporosis is responsible for more days spent in a hospital than diabetes, heart attacks and breast cancer.[11]

The burden to our healthcare system is staggering. Each year the U.S. spends nearly $17 billion treating more than two million osteoporotic fractures. When you add up the money spent in the United States, Canada and the European Union, $48 billion is spent every year treating osteoporotic fractures. This doesn't even consider the indirect costs such as disability, loss of productivity and the impacts on spouses and other family members.

**If you're a woman, your risk for breaking a bone because of osteoporosis is equal to your combined risk for breast, uterine and ovarian cancer. And if you're 50 years old or older, your risk of dying from a hip fracture is similar to your risk of dying from breast cancer.**

## Australia

In Australia, one third of women over 45 years old will develop osteoporosis. While more recent data aren't available, we know that in 2007 someone in Australia was admitted to a hospital with an osteoporotic fracture every 5-6 minutes.[12] That's worse than the next most recent data just six years earlier, so undoubtedly the situation is even more dire now.

## Asia

The number of people who are 60 years and over in Asian countries is predicted to triple between 2010 and 2050, reaching an estimated 1.3 billion by 2050.[13] Osteoporosis has become one of the most common and costly health problems in the region.[14]

Given the enormous aging population, it's not surprising that this region is expected to also experience a dramatic increase in hip fractures in the coming decades—half of all hip fractures in the world will occur in this region by 2050.[15] Over the past 30 years alone, the incidence of hip fractures have grown two- to three-times in most Asian countries.[16]

While getting older is a major driver of this increase, vitamin D deficiency, medications and diet are also important. In India, more than 80% of people are deficient in vitamin D. Similar to other regions around the world, like the Middle East, low sun exposure, inadequate consumption of vitamin D and calcium, lack of vitamin D food fortification, darker pigmented skin and a conservative dress code that has most of the skin covered may explain why vitamin D deficiency is so common.[17]

In Mainland China, a 2021 study determined that 5% of men and nearly 20% of women 40 years old and up have osteoporosis.[18] A previous study found that half of all women 80 years and older in Beijing have spinal fractures.[19] Similar to India and other Asian countries, low intake of vitamin D and calcium may partly explain how common osteoporosis is in China.

Many medications damage bone and cause osteoporosis and fractures. Glucocorticoids, which includes prednisone and dexamethasone, is one of the most powerful bone-destroying group of drugs. In India, 1% of adults are on long-term glucocorticoid therapy, which is a major contributing factor to the epidemic of osteoporosis in that country.[20]

## Europe

Europe's osteoporosis crisis is a tremendous burden to the European Union (EU). In 2019, the direct costs for treating fractures caused by osteoporosis was 36.3 billion Euros.[21] More than four million osteoporosis fractures occur each year in the EU, with about 75% of those occurring in just six countries—France, Germany, Italy, Spain, United Kingdom and Sweden.[22,23]

On the other hand, Portugal has one of the lowest fracture rates. Every year, there are an estimated 40,000 total osteoporotic fractures in Portugal, with 10,000 of those being hip fractures. And those numbers are going up. From 1989 to 2011, hip fractures increased by 81%—from 5,600 to 10,124.[24,25]

The cost for treating all these broken bones adds up. In 2011, for each patient who broke their hip the Portuguese government spent 13,434 euros during the first year and 5,985 euros in the second year after the fracture. In total, 216 million euros were spent in 2011 alone.[25] A little more than a decade later, there are now undoubtedly more fractures putting an even greater burden on Portugal's healthcare system.

## The Middle East

More than 80% of women in Middle Eastern countries are deficient in Vitamin D.[26] Since vitamin D is created when the sun hits the skin, the common practice in this region of covering most of the body year-round blocks vitamin D production. Additionally, due to the extreme heat, relatively more time is spent indoors compared to more temperate climates.

Death rates from osteoporosis in the Middle East are two to three times higher than in Western countries.[27] The International Osteoporosis Foundation (IOF) considers osteoporosis a "neglected" disease in the Middle East.

In Egypt alone, more than 80% of women have osteoporosis or osteopenia. Osteoporosis in Turkey is extremely common. Nearly 65% of men and women 65 years old or older have osteoporosis.[28]

Unfortunately, according to an IOF report published in 2012, the level of awareness among health care professionals is poor in many countries, and they are "ill-equipped to take care of patients with osteoporosis." In fact, at the time of their report, osteoporosis wasn't even integrated in the medical school education in most Middle Eastern countries except for Lebanon and Morocco.

Countries in the region with the highest rates of hip fractures include the United Arab Emirates (UAE), Jordan, Lebanon, Tunisia, Morocco, Syria, Saudi Arabia, Turkey and Iran. In Morocco, 50% of all postmenopausal women have vertebral fractures, and 60% of women with fractures have at least two.[27]

Unfortunately, most research into the causes of osteoporosis and fractures in this area of the world neglect to consider factors beyond vitamin D and calcium. As you'll learn later in this book, exercise, your overall dietary pattern, eating enough protein and adequate sleep are all crucial for bone health.

Clearly, if you wait for governments, medical societies and

insurance companies to synthesize the research and provide a holistic approach, it will be too late. You need to understand how you can take charge of your own health, strengthen your bones and reduce your fracture risk now. The first step to doing that is learning about your miraculous bones. Turn to the next chapter to get started.

## Chapter 3

# Miraculous Bones

When I was in medical school, we were taught that after bones reach their peak bone mass it's all downhill from there. During childhood and throughout puberty we build new bone faster than we lose it; therefore, bones become larger, denser and stronger. Women reach their peak bone density at about 22 years old, while men's bones continue to grow for about another five years.[1] But after that high point, the situation starts to reverse and people lose bone at 0.5% to 2% per year.[2] Estrogen helps build and maintain healthy bones, so in women the fastest period of bone loss happens when estrogen drops during menopause and the 10 years following.[3]

> Estrogen helps build and maintain healthy bones, so in women the fastest period of bone loss happens when estrogen drops during menopause and the 10 years following.

Bones are miracles of biological engineering. Like everything else in our bodies, they contain all the necessary machinery to thrive when we provide the right raw materials for them to do their job. The sad belief that bones are on this inevitable decline and there's nothing we can do about it is just plain wrong.

Our bones are not traveling down a hopeless one-way street of degeneration. As you'll learn in this book, if you give them what they need, bones can stay strong and healthy, and can even be regrown once you lose bone. But first, let's look at these self-regenerating miracles and all the ways they support us.

## Early Life

Bones begin their life early in pregnancy and are one of the first organs to start developing. By the second month, embryonic cells start differentiating into your spine and clavicle. After six weeks, an ultrasound shows arm and leg buds have developed, and by the end of the first trimester, your face, nose, fingers and toes become recognizable.

You're born with about 300 bones, but some of them fuse as you age. By the time you're an adult, there are about 206 individual bones left. Bones come in an impressive variety of shapes and sizes. There are flat bones like your sternum and most of the bones that make up your skull. Long bones like your femur in your thighs and humerus in your upper arms. Short bones that form your wrists and ankles. And irregular bones like your vertebrae. There isn't any other organ that has so many discrete parts scattered throughout your body.

Bones are incredibly strong. This makes it possible for you to stand, walk, run, drive a car, cook, chew food and hold your loved ones. Bones protect internal organs in the event of trauma and allow you to escape danger. A healthy spine can withstand hundreds of pounds of vertical loading (pressure pushing down) without breaking.[4]

## Why Bones are Strong

A bone's strength is the result of its unique composition. Bones are made up of two main components—minerals and collagen. Minerals, like calcium and magnesium, give bone its hardness. However, it's the collagen that gives bone its ultimate strength and provides the scaffolding that bind minerals.[5-8]

Collagen is made up of three strands of amino acids wrapped around each other. This creates an incredibly strong protein. To demonstrate this, my medical school histology professor, Richard Fredrickson, PhD, brought a chicken bone into the lab that he'd soaked in vinegar. Vinegar is a weak acid that dissolves minerals but leaves collagen behind. What you're left with is a bendable, rubbery bone. You can twist it, pull it, fold it in half; even bang it on a table or stomp on it and it won't break.

Collagen makes your bones flexible and supple enough to withstand a significant fall and not break. As you hit the ground, the force of the impact is dispersed through the bone. Healthy collagen absorbs the force of the fall, slightly bends and then returns to its original shape without a fracture.

However, without collagen, bones break easily. When you remove the collagen, the only thing left are the minerals. But minerals are brittle, like a piece of chalk. So for healthy, strong bones you need a combination of bone minerals and collagen.

Creating and maintaining both is the job of two cells: osteoblasts and osteoclasts. They're the workhorses of bone. Osteoblasts create new bone, and osteoclasts break down and recycle old bone in a process called bone remodeling. When your bones are growing, osteoblasts are working harder than osteoclasts. Once you hit peak bone mass and your bones are in a steady state—neither growing or decaying—the osteoblast and osteoclast activities are balanced. If you're losing bone, then your osteoclasts are more active than your osteoblasts. That's when you see your BMD test results going down and osteoporosis develops.

## Blood Factories

Your bones are more than minerals and collagen. Bones literally give you life. The spongy middle of bone is the marrow, which is a blood factory, taking nutrients and turning them into blood cells—red blood cells, white blood cells and platelets. Your red blood cells pick up oxygen from your lungs and deliver it to tissues and cells throughout your body. White blood cells fight infections and

> The spongy middle of bone is the marrow, which is a blood factory, taking nutrients and turning them into blood cells—red blood cells, white blood cells and platelets.

reduce your cancer risk. Platelets are required for healthy blood clotting. When you don't have enough platelets you can bruise more easily and experience life-threatening hemorrhages. If you have too many platelets, you can get dangerous blood clots. Platelets also store and release important molecules, including serotonin. You've likely heard of serotonin as one of your happy chemicals. Entire classes of medications have been developed that artificially increase serotonin as a treatment for depression. But most serotonin isn't in the brain at all. Cells in your intestines produce 95% of your body's serotonin, which never enters the brain. Instead, nearly all of the gut-derived serotonin is concentrated in platelets that circulate through your blood vessels.[9] All of those cells and their benefits are only possible because your bones create them.

## Bone as Part of the Endocrine System

Recent research has also revealed that bones create hormones. You've likely heard of melatonin's effects on sleep. It's produced by the pineal gland in the brain and helps you fall asleep. But just like serotonin, melatonin isn't only produced in the brain. Bone cells create melatonin and recent research has revealed melatonin as a powerful regulator of bone health.[10] Melatonin stimulates osteoblasts to create new bone. While this research is only just now emerging, one clinical trial has already shown that taking melatonin can improve BMD in postmenopausal women with osteoporosis.[10] I'll dive more into this research in Chapter 11, Dietary Supplements.

## Chapter 4

# Know Your Risks

O steoporosis is fundamentally a condition of imbalance. The destructive forces are winning, and it's your job to fight back, build stronger bones, increase your resilience and reestablish balance. One of the amazing things about life is that biological systems adapt to their environment. When you create the environment for your body to get stronger, it will.

This chapter is all about understanding threats to your health so you can take action to protect yourself. I identify risks that are in your control and those that aren't, so you know what to focus your time, energy and money on. Fortunately, you can change most of the risks.

But there are three important risks that you can't change. So let's get those out of the way first and put them in their proper perspective: your age, your personal medical history and your family's medical history.

The risk for osteoporosis and fractures increases as we get older. Although you can't magically make yourself younger,

> One of the amazing things about life is that biological systems adapt to their environment. When you create the environment for your body to get stronger, it will.

**Although you can't magically make yourself younger, you can turn back the clock by changing your diet and lifestyle, and by removing things from your life that damage bones.**

you can turn back the clock by changing your diet and lifestyle, and by removing things from your life that damage bones. You can improve how your biochemistry, cells and tissues function and improve your physiological age. That's why it's super important to take charge of your well being, be proactive and make your health your number one priority. After all, if you don't, who will?

In fact, a study of people 60 years and older showed that the greatest predictor for dying after a fracture isn't someone's age. It's whether they had other illnesses, such as a history of heart disease, mild or uncontrolled diabetes, chronic obstructive pulmonary disorder (COPD) or a liver disease. People with pre-existing conditions were 215% more likely to die within one year after breaking a hip compared to folks without other diseases. In comparison, simply getting older accounted for only a 3% increase in risk.[1] This just goes to show that being proactive and staying healthy pays off.

Yet even if you've already been diagnosed with other diseases, there's a lot you

**The greatest predictor for dying after a fracture isn't someone's age. It's whether they had other illnesses, such as a history of heart disease, mild or uncontrolled diabetes, chronic obstructive pulmonary disorder (COPD) or a liver disease.**

can do to control and even reverse them with diet and lifestyle changes. This is where working with a good integrative health-care provider—like a naturopathic doctor—can be extremely helpful.

When looking at your risks, a doctor will evaluate your medical and family history. For example, if you already had a previous osteoporosis fracture, you're automatically at greater risk for another one. Despite that, the research is clear: if you improve your strength and balance, you reduce your risk for falling, which automatically reduces your risk for breaking another bone.

If someone in your immediate family had osteoporosis or a hip fracture, it also automatically increases your risk. I've heard people—including doctors—say it's genetic, but that assumption has never been proven. First, bone health is determined by many genes. There isn't one "osteoporosis gene." More importantly, the research is clear that as we age the role of diet and lifestyle in the development of chronic diseases is much more important than your genes.

We know that genes by themselves don't really do anything. To become active and carry out their vital roles in health, they require a biochemical soup of nutrients, including water, vitamins, minerals, proteins, fats and phytochemicals (plant nutrients). At the most basic level, the role of genes is to create proteins, which include functional proteins like some hormones. Some examples are thyroid hormone, serotonin, dopamine, epinephrine and insulin. Proteins are also structural. Collagen is an example of a structural protein that, along with other proteins, make up bones, muscles, ligaments, tendons and more.

Lifestyle, diet and environmental toxin exposure are more important for long-term health than genetics. Research suggests that 80% of large bowel, breast and prostate cancers are caused by poor nutrition, physical inactivity and obesity.[2,3] And the predominant causes of heart disease and diabetes are the same—crappy diet, a sedentary lifestyle, sleep deprivation, chronic stress and obesity.

As you can see from the list of known risk factors in Table 1 below, genetics is not listed. But two other things you inherit from your parents are: diet and exercise. During childhood, food choices and exercise are largely based on your parent's preferences. Poor diet and exercise habits developed in childhood usually continue into adulthood, which increases the risk for osteoporosis and other chronic degenerative diseases.[4-6] The good news is that while there's nothing you can do about your past, you can reduce your risks if you're willing to put in the work.

**The good news is that while there's nothing you can do about your past, most of the risks can be reduced if you're willing to put in the work.**

**Table 1. Osteoporosis and Fracture Risks**

| | |
|---|---|
| Advanced age | Impaired vision |
| Caucasian race | Insomnia |
| Chronic stress | Low bone mineral density (BMD) |
| Current smoking, any amount | Low vitamin D intake |
| Dementia | Long-term low calcium intake |
| Depression | Low physical activity |
| Environmental hazards | More than two alcoholic drinks per day |
| Estrogen deficiency from early menopause (<45 years old) or having your ovaries removed | Poor health/frailty |
| Family history of osteoporosis | Poor nutrition |
| Going for more than one year without your period (amenorrhea) | Previous fracture (other than skull, facial bones, ankle, finger, or toe as an adult) |
| Having a disease that causes osteoporosis | Smoking |
| History of hip fracture in a parent | Taking a medication that causes osteoporosis and fracture |
| History of recent falls | Thinness (body weight < 127 lbs. [57.7 kg] or low BMI [<21 kg/m2]) |

One of the amazing things is that many of the risks are intertwined. When you improve in one area, it can also reduce your risks in other areas, and for the other illnesses. For example, getting your eyes checked is important for more than just your vision. If you have poor vision and can't enjoy things you used to love or are feeling socially isolated, that can create

> One of the amazing things is that many of the risks are intertwined. When you improve in one area, it can also reduce your risks in other areas, and for the other illnesses.

depression. Also, not being able to see well increases your risk for falling and breaking a bone.

Recommendations like cutting down on alcohol and quitting smoking are straightforward. If you're an alcoholic or addicted to nicotine, it may not be easy, but there are ample tried and true resources for you to tap into, like Alcoholics Anonymous or speaking to your doctor about smoking cessation programs. And when you surround yourself with people who support and encourage you, you're more likely to succeed and live healthier, which is one reason why Chapter 12 on Social Support is so important.

Proper nutrition and exercise reduce your risks because they combat depression, build muscle and increase strength and balance. But they also improve blood pressure, blood sugar and fasting insulin to reduce your heart disease and diabetes risks and are also associated with reducing dementia risk. Talk about some great side benefits! But what does eating right mean? And what are the best exercises? I walk you through all this in Chapters 7 and 8.

Medications are such a common and major risk that there's a chapter just for that too. If you take any medications—whether prescription or over the counter—it's crucial to know which ones cause osteoporosis and increase your fracture risk. When you read Chapter 5 you'll be shocked by the long list and how many doctors are unknowingly creating osteoporosis in their patients.

Sleep deprivation puts you at greater risk for falls and fractures, and insomnia has been associated with a 50% increase in the risk for osteoporosis.[7] I provide specific suggestions tailored to your needs in Chapter 10 to help you catch some ZZZ's.

But before we dive into all of that, here are some important, simple steps to take to make your home safer.

## Fracture-Proof Your Home

No one wants to feel unsafe in their home. But unfortunately, many falls occur in people's homes, so it's crucial to deal with dangers in the place you spend most of your time.

The North American Menopause Society (NAMS) recommends you:[8]

- fix loose steps and handrails that could cause you to lose your balance and fall
- get rid of throw rugs you could trip over
- keep walkways well lit
- clear furniture you could stumble over and fall
- add railings to your bathtub and toilet area

## Loose Steps and Handrails

Loose steps inside and outside the house are dangerous. They increase your risk for losing your balance and falling, even down an entire flight of stairs. In addition to fixing the steps, make sure handrails are solidly attached to the wall. Can you imagine how horrifying it would be to lose your balance and grab the handrail to save yourself, only to have it pull off the wall?

## Throw Rugs

Get rid of your throw rugs and fix loose carpet. It's easy to catch your foot on the edge of a throw rug or a piece of carpet that's slightly raised. They're particularly dangerous for people who shuffle as they walk. I've had too many patients fall and end up in the hospital precisely because of this hazard. That's what happened to my mother-in-law, Dee. A frequent shuffler, Dee once caught her foot on the edge of a throw rug, fell and broke her hip. Checking out and fixing what's on your floors is a no-brainer.

## Lighting

Make sure all common walkways are well lit, even throughout the night. If you get up in the middle of the night to go to the bathroom or head into the kitchen to get a drink of water, the hallway lights allow you to see anything you might trip over, such as the leg of a chair or corner of a table. You can purchase motion-detection lights that automatically switch on at night when you start walking near

**Make sure all common walkways are well lit, even throughout the night.**

them. They're inexpensive and battery operated, so you don't need an electrician or technical expertise. You can buy ones with adhesive backing that lets you simply stick them on a wall. You can also install lights that can be programmed to turn on at sundown or another time you choose and stay on all night.

## Clear Furniture and Other Obstructions

If you need more incentive to clean up clutter, osteoporosis is it! Make sure all walkways are clear of anything you can trip over, including boxes, unfinished projects and furniture. It's important to sacrifice attractive decorating for clear, wide walkways. When you're osteoporotic, even stubbing your toe could break a bone. Peggy, a 91-year-old retired teacher told me how she broke toes multiple times by bumping into furniture in her house.

The living room can be particularly hazardous. A low coffee table can be hard to navigate when you're groggy in the middle of the night, and a footstool in front of a couch can be difficult to see. And table corners can jut into walkways just enough to bump into them and fall.

## Secure Your Bathroom

The bathroom is a common area for slips and falls, especially for frail people with balance issues. Often people wake up in the middle of the night to pee. When you're groggy and a bit disoriented, it's a perfect combination for a disaster. Plus, when you take a sleep medication, your risk for falling is even higher.

In addition to removing throw rugs in your bathroom, including those in front of your sink, toilet and shower, put a slip-resistant bathmat in your shower or bathtub. Add grab bars wherever you're lifting a leg to step over something, or when the ground might be slippery or you're getting up from a seated position. The wall next to the toilet, in the bathtub and just outside the shower are good places for handrails. These bars will give you something to grab onto and maintain your balance or regain it in case you start to wobble.

## 🦴 Take Action 🦴

For those of you reading this who are super handy around the house, fixing up loose steps or adding handrails to your bathroom may be a snap. But for folks like me, it presents an insurmountable obstacle. My wife and kids have a running joke that when I pick up a hammer or drill, they know the expletives will follow.

In fact, I've put entire bookcases together and then realized that I've done it backwards or upside down and needed to take the whole thing apart and start over. But then again, people didn't show up to my medical clinical asking me to put a bookcase together. I am much better at helping people put their health back together.

If you can fracture-proof your house yourself, fantastic! If not, find someone to do it. You can search for a handyman through homeadvisor.com (I have no relationship with this company) or another company. Local service agencies such as Jewish Family Services (JFS), churches and community centers are great resources for finding help. If you're short on cash or on a fixed income, these organizations may be able to find donated materials and labor for you. Sometimes construction companies partner with service organizations to give back to their communities, and the nonprofit may have that help readily available for you.

Don't be intimidated to reach out to a religious organization even if you're not affiliated with them or even from their same religion. What I've found is that community service organizations of all types are filled with people who want to help their neighbors and their communities. So call your local house of worship or community center and ask if they can help, or if they can point you in the right direction to get you the help you need.

Before you tackle this project, however, it's important to know what needs to be done. To get the ball rolling, I'm providing a list of questions.

Your answers will help you get organized for doing the project yourself or will be needed when describing the job to someone else. You can also download and print this list at nbihealth.com/osteobook.

### Handrails and Steps

- Do you have loose steps?_____
- Loose handrails? _____
- Where? _____
- How many? _____
- What material are they (eg, wood, concrete)?

  _____

- Do you need help fixing any handrails or steps?

  _____

### Throw Rugs

- Do you have throw rugs in your home? _____
- Where? _____
- Do you need help getting rid of them? _____
- How will you get rid of them (eg, donate, store, sell, throw away)?_____

### Lighting

- Do you need more lighting along common walkways in your house? _____
- Where (eg, stairs, living room, hallway, etc.)?

  _____

- How many lights do you think you'll need (more is better)? _____
- Where will you purchase them? _____
- Do you need help buying or installing them?____

### Obstructions in Walkways

- Do walkways have furniture in them you can trip over or other obstructions? _____
- What type of furniture is it (eg, coffee table, end table, couch, chair, etc.)? _____
- How many pieces of furniture? _____
- Do you need help rearranging or getting rid of any furniture? _____

### Grab bars

• Are any existing grab bars loose and need to be tightened? _____

• How many bathrooms need new grab bars installed? _____

• How many total grab bars need to be installed?

_____

• How many existing grab bars need to be tightened? _____

• Do you need help fixing or installing grab bars?

_____

## Chapter 5

# The Danger in Your Medicine Cabinet

A mericans are some of the most medicated people in the world. In 2018 alone, nearly six billion prescriptions were filled, and more than two thirds of those were for just two illnesses—diabetes and hypertension.[1] According to the Centers for Disease Control and Prevention (CDC), about 50% of all Americans use at least one prescription drug, and doctors prescribe a medication in three quarters of all appointments.[2]

According to the Centers for Disease Control and Prevention (CDC), about 50% of all Americans use at least one prescription drug, and doctors prescribe a medication in three quarters of all appointments.

Not surprising, the older people get the more likely they are to take medications. In fact, 70% of adults age 40-79 are taking at least one prescription drug, which increases to 83% if you only count folks 60 years and older.[3]

And the number of medications increases with age too. In the United States, about 57% of women and 44% of men 65 years or older take at least five medications, and 12% take 10 or more.[4] Additionally, up to 91% of patients in long-term care facilities take five or more medications.[5]

While the over-use of medications is well-documented and shocking,[6] equally concerning is that doctors rarely talk to their patients about common and dangerous side effects. All medications come with risks, including nausea, drowsiness, dry mouth, rashes, diarrhea and serious complications such as liver damage or heart attacks and strokes. But too many people—including physicians—are ignorant of the dangerous effects common medications have on bone. These can include stripping bones of minerals, damaging collagen and increasing the risk for falls and fractures.[7]

Up to 30% of osteoporosis cases in postmenopausal women come from external causes, such as medications, instead of the drop in estrogen that comes with menopause.[8] And in premenopausal women and men it's up to a staggering 50%.[9-11]

> Up to 30% of osteoporosis cases in postmenopausal women come from external causes, such as medications, instead of the drop in estrogen that comes with menopause. And in premenopausal women and men it's up to a staggering 50%.

Medications that damage bone include glucocorticoids, such as prednisone and dexamethasone, acid blockers, anticoagulants, antidepressants, diabetes drugs, blood pressure medications and medications commonly used for cancer, endometriosis and uterine fibroids.

Other medications increase the risk for falls because

they create dizziness, drowsiness, confusion, blurred vision or make you lightheaded when you stand up. Those culprits are prescribed for common conditions, such as anxiety, insomnia, high blood pressure, tight muscles and even some medications for allergies and memory loss. Taking multiple medications increases your risk for falls and being hospitalized and—shockingly—95% of people 65 years or older are prescribed a medication that increases their risk for falling.[12,13] Some drugs even do both—weaken bones and increase falls.

**Shockingly, 95% of people 65 years or older are prescribed a medication that increases their risk for falling.**

If you're on medications that damage bone or increase your fall risk, it might be possible to lower the dose of the medication, switch to a safer one, or discontinue it all together. But I caution you not to simply trust your doctor will switch you to a safer one. A study looked at the medications patients were taking in the four months before and after they broke a bone, and the results were shocking.

Prior to the fracture, 42% of patients were taking at least one medication that decreased bone density, 76% were on at least one medication known to increase fracture risk, and about 56% were taking at least one medication that increased the risk for falling. One would think that after the patient broke a bone their doctor would switch them to a safer medication. Unfortunately, less than half of the patients taking bone-damaging and fracture-creating medications were taken off those drugs.[14]

**Prior to the fracture, 42% of patients were taking at least one medication that decreased bone density, 76% were on at least one medication known to increase fracture risk, and about 56% were taking at least one medication that increased the risk for falling.**

For most types of medications such as antidepressants, acid blockers and medications for insomnia and anxiety, 75-94% of the time the doctors didn't switch the medications. And nearly 11% of patients who weren't taking one of the dangerous medications before they broke a bone were put on one after. How insane is that? You break a bone and then the doctor puts you on a medication that increases your risk to beak another bone. The saddest part of all is that these doctors likely don't even realize this mistake because most of them don't understand how common the problem is.

In this chapter I review some of the most prescribed medications. If you're taking any medication listed in Table 1, make sure to talk to your doctor and pharmacist. The table lists categories of medications, and within those categories are hundreds of different drugs. While your doctor might not know the risk off the top of her head, perhaps she'll look it up. But don't rely solely on your doctor.

While physicians are knowledgeable about prescribing and managing medications, pharmacists are *the experts* and one of the most underutilized healthcare professionals.

They're incredibly smart and well-educated, yet most spend their days solely filling prescriptions. They not only know the most about medications, but they can also easily access the most up-to-date databases of potential side effects. Get to know your local pharmacist and ask them questions about your medications.

If you can't stop taking the medication, then you really need to be doing everything possible to protect yourself. This includes following my Osteoporosis Diet, exercising appropriately, getting enough sleep and supplementing with the right nutrients. I discuss all of this in detail in later chapters, and my supplement recommendations are generally the right ones for most people. Where medications have effects that require more specific recommendations, I provide those in the suggestions below.

**Table 1. Drugs that Damage Bones or Increase Falls**

| |
| --- |
| Acid-blocking medications |
| Aluminum-coated antacids |
| Androgen deprivation therapy (ADT) |
| Antidepressants |
| Antihistamines |
| Antipsychotics |
| Anxiety meds (Benzodiazepines)* |
| Blood pressure meds |

(cont.)

| |
|---|
| Chemotherapy |
| Depot medroxyprogesterone acetate |
| Diabetes meds |
| Epilepsy meds |
| Excessive thyroid hormone |
| Glucocorticoids |
| Heparin |
| Immunosuppressants |
| Lithium |
| Memory meds (Anticholinergics) |
| Muscle relaxants |
| Opioids |
| Sleep meds (sedative hypnotics)* |

*These drugs are commonly prescribed for anxiety and sleep. They include Sonata, Lunesta, Halcion, Belsomra, ProSom, Versed and more.

Before I talk about solutions in more detail, I want you to have a good understanding of what these medications do to people. You'll undoubtedly want to talk to your doctor about this, so it's important to be armed with the facts. First, you may not need your medication at all. A 2020 study that looked at medications prescribed to people 65 years old and older determined that more than one-third of those prescriptions were potentially inappropriate.[15]

Additionally, there are effective integrative and natural ways to work with patients with chronic diseases that give results without medications, or that allow us to reduce the dose or number of medications people are taking. When considering your options, consider working with a naturopathic or functional doctor. They're trained to look for the underlying causes of symptoms and to treat people with nutrition-

> A 2020 study that looked at medications prescribed to people 65 years old and older determined that more than one-third of those prescriptions were potentially inappropriate.

al, lifestyle and holistic approaches instead of reflexively prescribing a medication.

## Glucocorticoids

This category of medications includes prednisone and dexamethasone. They go by such names as Deltasone, Prednicot, Prednisone Intensol, Sterapred, Baycadron Elixe, Decadron, Dekpak 13 Day Taperpak, Dexamethasone Intensol, DexPak, DexPak 10 Day TaperPak and Zema-Pak.

Glucocorticoids powerfully suppress inflammation and modulate the immune system. Short-term and long-term prescriptions are commonly used to treat autoimmune and inflammatory diseases, including rheumatoid arthritis (RA), polymyalgia rheumatic, asthma, irritable bowel disease (IBD), rashes and chronic obstructive pulmonary disease (COPD).

These medications are so popular that an estimated 1-2% of the general population are taking them long-term, meaning for months and years.[16] And in specific subpopulations that number is higher. Nearly 5% of women with postmenopausal osteoporosis—who definitely should try to avoid medications that weaken bones—are on these drugs.[17,18]

Nearly 5% of women with postmenopausal osteoporosis—who definitely should try to avoid medications that weaken bones—are on these drugs.

Glucocorticoids are so dangerous that fractures occur in up to 50% of patients who take them long-term.[19] They're such potent bone destroyers that even taking a low dose—less than 2.5 mg/day over just six months—increases fracture risk up to 200% compared to patients not taking them.[20] And one study found that every time a patient's dose increases by as little as 10 mg, their fracture risk increases by a whopping 62%.[21]

Glucocorticoids are so dangerous that fractures occur in up to 50% of patients who take them long-term.

Until recently it was generally accepted that only people chronically taking the drugs (for months or longer) were at risk. But we now know that even taking them for as little as six days can cause problems. A 2017 study debunked the assumption that short-term glucocorticoid use is safe. People who took these medications had an 87% higher chance of breaking a bone compared to people who hadn't taken the medication.[22]

These drugs damage bone both directly and indirectly. They directly decrease osteoblast activity while increasing osteoclasts, which you now know is bad. The drugs impact bone indirectly because they affect the nervous system and your hormones, alter the way calcium is processed, reduce collagen production and damage muscle. This results in bones losing minerals and collagen, and weaker muscles. This increases your risk of falling, and since your bones are also now weaker, your risk for fractures is scary high. Fortunately, after discontinuing the glucocorticoids, fracture risk declines. However, we don't know whether your bones will ever get back to their pre-medication strength.[20,23-25]

One of the challenges in helping patients who are taking glucocorticoids is that fracture risk increases before we can detect changes in BMD.[21] Essentially, this means that even if your bone density is normal, you and your doctor should still assume that damage is occurring. Even with this limitation, I recommend patients get a bone density test before starting long-term glucocorticoid treatment, and then track their bone health with follow up bone density testing.

## Acid Blockers

Reducing stomach acid is frequently recommended to treat gastroesophageal reflux disorder (known as GERD, acid reflux and heartburn), erosive esophagitis, a *Helicobacter pylori* (*H. pylori*) stomach infection and ulcers. Acid blocking drugs are big business. They're one of the most widely prescribed drugs in the world, raking in $11 billion in sales every year.[26] In the U.S., more than 15 million patients receive 157 million prescriptions a year of only one type of acid blocker called proton pump inhibitors.[27]

Half of all prescriptions are to treat acid reflux, which is incredible since heartburn is mainly a condition caused by poor diet.[28] Unfortunately, just like with osteoporosis, doctors are more likely to prescribe a pill than to have a longer, more involved conversation about diet and lifestyle. If you've got acid reflux, first try eliminating the seven common food triggers and you might see your symptoms disappear. They are tomato and tomato products, raw garlic, raw onion, coffee, chocolate, citrus and spicy foods. Through trial and error, you can add one food back at a time and see which ones causes you problems.

Acid blockers have consistently been shown to increase falls and fracture risk. I'm sure you've heard of these drugs as the ads are all over television and in magazines, and they've been available without a prescription since 2003. They come in two types based on how they suppress your stomach acid. Proton pump inhibitors (PPIs) include esomeprazole (Nexium), omeprazole (Prilosec, "the little purple pill"), pantoprazole (Protonix), lansoprazole (Prevacid) and rabeprazole (Aciphex). The other type blocks histamine production. These include famotidine (Pepcid) and cimetidine (Tagamet) and are referred to as H2 receptor antagonist (H2RA) meds.

Both types of acid blockers increase fracture risk. In 2010 the FDA warned that PPIs increase the risk for hip, spine or lower arm (radius bone) fractures.[29] The earliest study that looked at this issue goes all the way back to 2006 when researchers determined that taking any type of acid blocker increases fracture risk up to 82% compared to people not taking them.[30]

Like glucocorticoids and other medications, the longer someone takes the medication and the higher the dose, the greater the danger. Even though the FDA has never approved these drugs for long-term use—especially for acid reflux—in the real-world people take them for years. Of the two types of acid blocking medications, PPIs seem to be the most dangerous. After four years of taking PPIs, the risk for a hip fracture increases to 217% compared to people not taking the meds. When their analysis was restricted to patients with only heartburn, the risk for fractures from PPIs was even worse —350% greater risk.[30]

Not only do PPIs weaken bones, they also increase the risk for falling. A 2019 analysis of data from more than 350,000 patients determined that PPIs increased the risk for falling by 27%, and the risk of a fall that resulted in hospitalization by 61%.[31]

If you're on an acid-blocker and lose bone, your doctors will probably recommend one of the FDA-approved osteoporosis medications. This has been the standard of care in conventional osteoporosis treatment for years. The most prescribed osteoporosis medications are the bisphosphonates (Fosamax, Actonel, Boniva and Reclast), and those are likely what you'd get.

But a 2015 study threw cold water on that approach. Bisphosphonates don't reduce fractures in these patients. In fact, they do the exact opposite; they create more fractures. Data from nearly 60,000 patients showed that combining a PPI with any type of bisphosphonate increased fractures by 52% compared to patients who only took a bisphosphonate.[32] None of the other types of osteoporosis medications have been studied in people taking acid-blocking drugs, so we don't know if they'd help. However, before taking a medication, it's important to make sure it's appropriate and can help. In the next chapter, I discuss this in detail and provide questions to ask your doctor and pharmacist.

PPIs increase fracture risk by causing nutritional deficiencies, including magnesium, calcium and vitamin B12. Decreased magnesium increases bone breakdown while slowing the creation of new bone. Bones are the body's reservoir for calcium. When there isn't enough calcium in the blood, your body increases a hormone called parathyroid hormone (PTH). When that happens your bones release calcium into the blood, and over time this can cause osteoporosis.

One study found that both vitamin B12 and serum ferritin significantly decreased after just one year of taking a PPI while another one found that after three years of taking the medication, 22.2% were deficient in vitamin B12.[33,34] Low vitamin B12 can lead to bone destruction by increasing a damaging protein in the blood called homocysteine. And if that weren't enough, low vitamin B12 can cause loss of muscle strength and numbness and tingling in your hands and feet, a situation called peripheral neuropathy. Decreased muscle strength and peripheral neuropathy increase your risk for falling and breaking a bone.

Ferritin is the storage form of iron, and a serum ferritin test is the most sensitive and reliable indicator for iron status.[35-38] Your doctor likely won't order this test without being asked, so ask for a serum ferritin test or order your own online. One challenge, however, is interpreting the results. Normal reference ranges can vary by lab, and serum ferritin levels from 12 to 200 nanograms per milliliter (ng/mL) are often considered normal.[39]

However, iron deficiency is likely when the ferritin level falls below 50 ng/mL. A large study of nearly 200 women ages 18-53 years confirms that iron supplementation should begin long before a person's serum ferritin becomes "abnormal." When women in the study had a ferritin below 50 and they complained of fatigue, they were given an iron supplement. When they took the iron supplement for three months their energy increased by nearly 50%.[40] Another study reported benefit from taking iron when ferritin was less than 50 nanograms per milliliter in people with restless leg syndrome (RLS).[41]

Most doctors will look at the test result—even when it's down to 20 or 30—and say, "You're in the normal range so you're fine." But normal does not mean optimal, and you want optimal levels of essential nutrients. People's serum ferritin should be above 50 ng/mL, and I prefer my patients get closer to 90 to 110.

If you need extra iron, FerroSolve is the product I created for my patients after hearing repeated complaints of cramping, constipation and nausea from other iron dietary supplements. FerroSolve contains a unique form of iron that is highly absorbable and promotes healthy iron levels without upsetting your gastrointestinal system.

Since vitamin B12 and magnesium aren't toxic, it's probably a good idea to supplement with those and other B vitamins and minerals that acid blockers might affect. Look for a high-quality multiple vitamin and mineral supplement that contains methylfolate (the biologically active form of folic acid) and magnesium as magnesium glycinate, magnesium citrate or magnesium as an amino acid chelate. Those forms of magnesium will be the best absorbed.

Currently there aren't any published guidelines for the prevention or treatment of osteoporosis caused by acid blocking medications. Given the evidence, taking acid blocking medications short-term, perhaps for a couple of weeks, is likely safe. But people should try to avoid taking them for long periods of time. If they can be avoided altogether, even better. If you're taking an acid blocking medication because of heartburn, there are great resources on the NBI website that provide natural approaches you can try. Go to nbihealth.com and search "acid reflux."

## Antidepressants

Antidepressants are popular, widely used drugs. Almost 14% of all US adults took antidepressants in 2018, and that was before the pandemic turned everyone's world upside down. Like with so many other things, the older people get, the greater the risk for depression. Nearly 25% of all women 60 years old and older took an antidepressant in 2018.[42]

There are different types of antidepressants. They're categorized based on how they act in the body. The most-prescribed antidepressants are the selective serotonin reuptake inhibitors (SSRIs) and serotonin-norepinephrine reuptake inhibitors (SNRIs). Serotonin is considered one of our "happy chemicals," and these drugs artificially boost serotonin. Doctors not only prescribe them for depression, but also for anxiety disorders, premenstrual syndrome, chronic pain, fibromyalgia, peripheral neuropathy, and menopausal hot flashes.

The SSRI medications go by such names as citalopram (Celexa), escitalopram (Lexapro), fluoxetine (Prozac), paroxetine (Paxil), sertraline (Zoloft). The SNRIs are atomoxetine (Strattera), desvenlaxafine (Pristiq), duloxetine (Cymbalta) and venlaxafine (Effexor XR). You've likely seen some commercials for these medications on television, with cheerful music and eye-catching images to entice you to ask your doctor to prescribe one for you. The quickly read, long list of side effects are easy to ignore. But even in their list of side effects, I've never heard them mention osteoporosis. They should.

In a Canadian study that tracked patients for 10 years, researchers found that taking either an SSRI or an SNRI was associated with a 68% increase in fracture risk.[43] Another study found that women taking SSRIs were losing bone more than 1.6 times faster than women who weren't on those meds.[44]

> Taking either an SSRI or an SNRI was associated with a 68% increase in fracture risk.

Two studies evaluated how many patients would have to take SSRIs before one of them experienced a fracture. One of the studies determined your gender or age didn't matter; the fracture risk was the same.[45] For every 42 patients taking an SSRI, we can expect one of them will break their hip, wrist or forearm. The researchers working on the second study evaluated their data a little differently. They looked at the risk for fractures based on how long someone took the medicine. They found that even taking an SSRI for just a year or less still increased someone's fracture risk so much that for every 85 patients taking the medication, they'd expect one of them to break a bone.

It got even worse the longer someone took the drug. For every 19 patients taking the antidepressant for one to five years, one of them would be expected to break a bone.[46] This is extremely alarming since nearly 25 million adults have been on antidepressants for more than two years. Another 15.5 million have been on the medications for at least five years, and many people find it extremely difficult to discontinue these medications because of the side effects they experience when they try to do so.[47]

> For every 19 patients taking the antidepressant for one to five years, one of them would be expected to break a bone.

Most people, including doctors, aren't aware that serotonin has powerful effects on bones. When people artificially increase their serotonin with these drugs, it indirectly damages bone by altering the nervous system, which increases the activity of bone-destroying osteoclasts. And they directly damage bones by decreasing the activity of bone-building osteoblasts. With a natural balance of serotonin, you get strong bones because the effects of bone-destroying osteoclasts are offset by osteoblasts.

But these medications throw off that delicate balance, which damages bones, causes osteoporosis and creates fractures. There are no published guidelines on preventing or treating bone loss caused by antidepressants. I recommend patients taking these medications get a bone density test before starting them, and then at regular intervals to monitor their bones. Additionally, since underlying nutritional deficiencies are associated with depression, testing for these nutrients may determine if you need extra. Nutrient deficiencies associated with depression include vitamins B3, B6, B12 and folic acid,[48-50] iron and magnesium,[51] and the amino acids L-tryptophan, phenylalanine, tyrosine and methionine.[52-54] Treatment plans based on this approach have been shown to alleviate depression and may provide the opportunity to reduce or discontinue the antidepressant medication.[55]

## Aromatase Inhibitors

Bone loss in women with breast cancer is a major concern. Up to 80% of all breast cancer patients lose bone.[56,57] Plus, breast cancer patients who are hospitalized with a fracture have an 83% higher risk of dying compared to breast cancer patients who don't break a bone.[58]

> Up to 80% of all breast cancer patients lose bone. Plus, breast cancer patients who are hospitalized with a fracture have an 83% higher risk of dying compared to breast cancer patients who don't break a bone.

About 80% of breast cancers get worse when there's estrogen in the body. This is called estrogen receptor-positive

(ER-positive) breast cancer. Aromatase inhibitors (AIs) block estrogen production and are one of the top-prescribed drugs for postmenopausal women with this type of cancer.[59,60] Once a woman is taking an AI, it's common for her to take it for many years. These medications go by such names as exemestane (Aromasin), letrozole (Femara) and anastrozole (Arimidex).

As I mentioned in Chapter 3, the fastest rate of bone loss occurs during menopause and for ten years after. But taking AIs increases that bone loss up to four times faster. This rapid bone loss increases the risk for osteoporosis and fractures. After five years of taking an AI, one in every five patients—an alarming 20%—breaks a bone.[61]

**After five years of taking an AI, one in every five patients—an alarming 20%—breaks a bone.**

By suppressing estrogen, AIs create a cascade of events that increase reactive oxygen species (ROS), which are involved in inflammation and damaging cells and tissues, and create an unhealthy microenvironment in bones.[62] Because of that and other effects, estrogen deficiency caused by AIs not only increases osteoclast formation, but also increases how long osteoclasts hang around and destroy bones. The result is rapid bone loss and increased risk of fracture.

Even though the National Comprehensive Cancer Network (NCCN) and the American Society for Clinical Oncology (ASCO) recommend all breast cancer patients taking an AI get bone density tests, many don't. Only about 42% to 68% of all women starting this treatment get a bone density test.[63-67] So make sure you ask for a bone density test and track your bone health with repeat testing.

Bisphosphonates and another osteoporosis medication—denosumab (Prolia)—have been studied in people taking AIs. In postmenopausal women with ER-positive breast cancer, bisphosphonates increased bone density, but haven't been shown to prevent fractures. Denosumab has been shown to reduce fractures by 50% and is therefore the better choice. [61]

## Androgen-Deprivation Therapy

Androgen-deprivation therapy (ADT) is used in women to treat polycystic ovarian syndrome (PCOS), endometriosis, uterine myomas and premenopausal breast cancer. In men, physicians prescribe ADT to treat prostate cancer. Medications include leuprolide (Lupron, Eligard), goserelin (Zoladex), triptorelin (Trelstar) and histrelin (Vantras, Supprelin LA).

Premenopausal women who take an ADT drug are put into a chemically induced menopause, which increases their risk for bone loss and fractures.[68] In men and women, these drugs create osteoporosis by increasing inflammation and stimulating osteoclasts to dissolve more bone.[69,70] Bone loss has been detected in patients as young as 29 years old after only three months of ADT treatment.[71] But there's another dangerous effect with ADT that we don't see with AIs. The loss of testosterone (in men and women) leads to muscle wasting, decreased strength and increased risk for falls and fractures.[72]

In men undergoing prostate cancer treatment, within one year of starting an ADT medication, they lose about 5% of their bone mass.[73] The story with this medication is the same as other meds—the longer the drug is taken, the worse the damage. In one

**In one study of men with prostate cancer taking an ADT drug, 43% got osteoporosis after two years, 50% after four years and 81% after 10 years.**

study of men with prostate cancer taking an ADT drug, 43% got osteoporosis after two years, 50% after four years and 81% after 10 years.[74]

And what about fractures? The risk for any fracture in men was 21%, and 30% for a hip fracture compared to men not taking the medication.[75] The older the man, the greater their risk. In men 81-85 years old there was a 42% increase and in men older than 85, there was a 48% increase in fracture risk compared to younger men 61-71 years old. Similar to women taking an AI, one study found that nearly 20% of men who were treated with ADT for prostate cancer and survived had broken a bone five years later.[76]

**Nearly 20% of men who were treated with ADT for prostate cancer and survived had broken a bone five years later.**

There are some things patients can do to reduce their risk. If you're a woman being treated for endometriosis, clinical guidelines recommend taking the ADT medication for no longer than six months, followed by add-back hormone therapy.[77] If you're a man undergoing prostate cancer treatment, you should get a bone density test before starting ADT and at regular intervals during treatment, exercise regularly to promote strength and balance and take calcium and vitamin D.[78]

These guidelines are lacking in two respects. First, consuming enough protein is crucial for preventing and reversing sarcopenia (muscle wasting), which makes people weaker, decreases balance and increases your risk for falls and fractures. I provide specific recommendations for protein in Chapter 7.

Second, people should consider taking MK4 based on the results of a six month, randomized clinical trial that showed taking 45 mg/day of MK4 (alone and in combination with vitamin D3) supported healthy bone density in women being treated with ADT.[79] In Chapter 11, I review these and other bone-support nutrients in more detail.

**Take Action**

Check all your medication, both prescription and over-the-counter. While you can do that here in the book, I created a sheet you can download and print to make it easier for you to show your doctor and pharmacist. You can download and print it at nbi-health.com/osteobook.

**Write down all your medications that are listed in Table 1.**

_____

_____

_____

_____

_____

_____

_____

**Write down all your medications not listed in Table 1.**

_____

_____

_____

_____

_____

_____

Call your doctor and request a medication review. Before your appointment, take all your medications to your local pharmacy and ask your pharmacist to check if any of the medications cause osteoporosis or increase your risk for falls or fractures. This will give you a list of medications of concern to bring to your appointment.

## Chapter 6

# Osteoporosis Meds 101

Learning you have osteoporosis is overwhelming. Every patient who has come to me with this diagnosis had been prescribed an osteoporosis medication. I've had patients report that their doctors emphatically told them—with 100% certainty—that if they didn't take the medication, they'd break a bone. One doctor even said he wouldn't work with a patient if she didn't take the drug.

The goal of every doctor should be to provide the best possible information so patients can make the best decision for themselves. A simple concept all healthcare providers learn is *informed consent*. This means you—the patient—have been told the potential benefits, risks and alternatives and you've had an opportunity to get your questions answered. You deserve to have all your questions answered and concerns addressed, so it's particularly upsetting to me that patients sometimes feel pressured into making a decision.

If you don't remember anything else from this chapter, remember this: While a diagnosis of osteopenia or osteoporosis may be scary, it's not an emergency. When you understand this, hopefully you'll take a deep breath, take some time to evaluate your options and put a holistic bone-building plan together. Perhaps a medication will be part of your plan, but maybe it won't. Ultimately, it's your decision whether or not to take a drug.

Additionally, conversations with healthcare providers usually focus solely on improving bone density. I've said this before, but it's so important that it bears repeating. The number on the test is not the most dangerous thing about osteoporosis. The most dangerous thing is breaking a bone, and that's what doctors are trying to prevent with treatments. Therefore, any intervention is only as valuable as it's been shown to reduce fractures.

Prescribing a medication is a judgment call. The clinician is saying she believes (1) the medication is appropriate, (2) the medication will help you and (3) the potential benefits outweigh the risks. And she may be right. But too often I've seen patients on medications they should never have been prescribed because the science simply doesn't justify it.

Let's say you get screened, and your doctor believes a medication is needed. By asking a few simple questions, it can help you understand whether the drug is appropriate and something you'll be comfortable taking. I'll walk you through what the research shows and what I think is the best way for healthcare providers to talk to their patients.

I won't review the details of every medication. That would take an entire book. Instead, this chapter gives you a checklist of questions to ask so you can make your decision based on facts instead of fear.

## Lots of Options

In 2020 the global osteoporosis market was valued at more than $13 billion. As you might imagine, with a market that big drug manufacturers have created lots of options to address the need. There are at least a dozen different drugs divided into two broad categories. Those that reduce bone breakdown are called antiresorptive medications. Those that build bone are called anabolic medications.

### The antiresorptive medications include:

- Bisphosphonates: alendronate (Fosamax), ibandronate (Boniva), risedronate (Actonel), and zoledronic acid (Zometa). These are taken orally either daily or weekly, except for Zometa, which is given intravenously every 12-18 months.
- Monoclonal antibody drugs: denosumab (Xgeva, Prolia). These are taken by an injection just under the skin every six months.
- Natural hormones: calcitonin, estrogen. Calcitonin is taken daily as a nasal spray, while estrogen is typically taken daily by mouth or absorbed through the skin with a patch.
- Estrogen modifiers: raloxifene (Evista), tamoxifen, toremifene (Fareston) change how estrogen acts in the body and are taken daily by mouth.

**The anabolic medications include:**

- Parathyroid hormone (PTH): teriparatide (Forteo).
  This is taken by subcutaneous injection once a day.
- Parathyroid hormone related peptide (PTHrP):
  abaloparatide (Tymlos). This is taken by subcutaneous
  injection once a day.
- Monoclonal antibody: romosozumab (Evenity)—
  approved in 2017—is the first new drug in about 15
  years and is taken by subcutaneous injection twice
  a month.

With so many options, how can you evaluate which one, if
any, might be a good fit? Simply put, a medication should be
appropriate for:

- your diagnosis
- your fracture history
- the bones you're trying to protect
- your risk tolerance
- your level of commitment

## Your Diagnosis

The most common osteoporosis diagnosis is postmenopausal
osteoporosis. It's important to note, however, that up to 30%
of osteoporosis cases in postmenopausal women come from
causes other than solely the drop in estrogen that happens
with menopause.[1] And in premenopausal women and men

it's up to 50%.[2-4] Medications, like those discussed in Chapter 5, and chronic diseases are two common secondary causes of osteoporosis.

If your doctor hasn't evaluated your medications or other diagnoses and whether they can be causing your problem, this needs to be done before you're sent off with another prescription. If a medicine is causing your osteoporosis and you're able to lower the dose, discontinue it or switch to a safer one, then you're well on your way to helping your bones heal.

When your doctor recommends an osteoporosis medication, ask if it's been shown in clinical trials to prevent fractures in people on the same medication (eg, your antidepressant, acid-blocker, glucocorticoid, etc.) or with the same disease that created your osteoporosis. As I discussed in Chapter 5, in medication-induced osteoporosis bone becomes damaged in different ways depending on the drug you're taking; therefore, it's difficult to accurately generalize the results from a study on one drug and apply it to a different one.

> **If your doctor hasn't evaluated your medications or other diagnoses and whether they can be causing your problem, this needs to be done before you're sent off with another prescription.**

## Your Fracture History

In addition to knowing if the drug prevents fractures in someone with your diagnosis, you also must know if it prevents fractures in people with your fracture history. A previous osteoporosis fracture is one of the strongest predictors for a future break. For women 65-74 years old with osteoporosis, the research shows that if you break a bone there's a 10% chance that you'll break another bone within a year, an 18% chance within two years and 31% chance you'll break another bone within five years. Women 75 years and older are at even greater risk. Research shows that 42% will break another bone within five years.[5]

If you've never had an osteoporosis fracture, the goal is primary fracture prevention. This is medicine's way of saying we're trying to prevent you from breaking a bone in the first place. If you already had a fracture and we're trying to prevent a subsequent one, it's called secondary fracture prevention. Therefore, it's important to ask your doctor if the medication has been shown in clinical trials to prevent primary fractures, secondary fractures or both.

**It's important to ask your doctor if the medication has been shown in clinical trials to prevent primary fractures, secondary fractures or both.**

Doctors often talk about "fractures" as if all bones are the same. This suggests a drug that prevents fractures in one part of the body does so throughout the body. Intuitively, it makes sense. A bone is a bone, so if one bone is protected, they're all protected, right? Wrong.

Body weight and movement put different stresses on bones. As a result, some fractures are more common than others.

Only 27% of osteoporosis fractures occur in the spine, while 73% occur elsewhere such as your hips or wrists.[6] Despite that, the vast majority of studies that report fractures only discuss vertebral fracture risk. That's because even when the drugs reduce spine fractures, they're less effective at preventing hip fractures. In addition to asking whether the medication is for primary or secondary fracture prevention, you also then need to ask if the drug has been shown in clinical trials to prevent both spinal fractures *and* hip fractures.

Similarly, when doctors focus solely on improving bone density, people might think they're protected when they're not. All FDA-approved medications improve bone density, so doctors feel good about the job they've done, and patients feels safe. But feeling safe and being safe are two different things. A medication may reduce vertebral fracture risk without reducing your risk of hip or other fractures. To be as protected as possible, ideally the drug will reduce spine and hip fractures. See Table 1.

A 2020 study that evaluated data from 22 different studies concluded that oral bisphosphonates only prevent fractures in people who had already had one. The medications do not prevent primary hip fractures.[7] An even larger study looking

**Oral bisphosphonates do not prevent primary fractures.** at 57 clinical trials with more than 100,000 postmenopausal women came to the same conclusion.[8] Despite that, these medications are what nearly all doctors recommend first to their patients!

In contrast to oral bisphosphonates, the intravenous bisphosphonate Zometa reduces primary vertebral fractures by 54% and primary non-vertebral fractures (wrist, arm, hip) by 33% in postmenopausal women with osteoporosis. None of the other categories of medications reduce the risk for primary vertebral and non-vertebral fractures.[8]

If you've already broken a bone, medications are more effective at preventing another fracture. In those cases, Tymlos, Fosamax, Boniva, Prolia, Actonel, Evenity, Forteo and Zometa decrease the risk for secondary vertebral and nonvertebral fractures.[8]

## Which Bones?

Understanding which bones you're trying to protect is crucial because some medications prevent secondary vertebral fractures, but not nonvertebral fractures. If you have a spinal fracture, taking a medication that reduces vertebral fractures—even if it doesn't prevent other fracture types, may still be a good option. For example, calcitonin reduces secondary vertebral fractures but not hip fractures. It can also reduce bone pain.[10] Evista also reduces secondary vertebral fractures but not hip fractures. Because of the nuances of the different medications, it's important to have this discussion with your doctor. The Take Action section, below, will help you organize your questions before your appointment.

**Table 1. Prevention of both Vertebral *and* Non-vertebral Fractures in Postmenopausal Osteoporosis**[8,10,11]

| Medication | Primary Prevention | Secondary Prevention |
|---|---|---|
| Fosamax (alendronate) | No | Yes |
| Boniva (ibandronate) | No | Yes |
| Actonel (risedronate) | No | Yes |
| Zometa (zoledronate) | Yes | Yes |
| Prolia (denosumab) | No | Yes |
| Calcitonin | No | No |
| Evista (reloxifene) | No | No |
| Forteo (parathyroid hormone) | No | Yes |
| Evenity (romosozumab) | No | Yes |
| Tymlos (apaloparatide) | No | Yes |

## Your Risk Tolerance

If you decide a medication might help, then you also need to understand the potential risks. With medications we're always balancing potential benefits with potential harm. Ask your doctor and pharmacist about the risks and the probability that you might experience any of them.

For example, according to the FDA package insert for

Zometa, more than 25% of patients experience nausea, fatigue, anemia, bone pain, constipation, fever, vomiting and shortness of breath. That may be an acceptable risk for you, especially if the goal is secondary fracture prevention. But without knowing the risk, how can you make an informed decision?

In a sad irony, oral bisphosphonates can create weaker bones and increase someone's fracture risk.[12,13] When a bisphosphonate causes a fracture, it's called an *atypical fracture*, and the risk increases the longer someone takes the medication. In one study that looked at this issue, after four or more years of taking an oral bisphosphonate, the risk for an atypical fracture was 0.1%.[14] This translates into one atypical fracture for every 1,000 people taking the drug for four or more years.

Bisphosphonate-related osteonecrosis of the jaw (BRONJ) happens when your jawbone gets damaged and can't heal. Most often this occurs during a dental procedure, like getting a tooth pulled. The exposed jawbone can become infected and begin to die. It's a dangerous and very difficult situation to treat.

**The risk for BRONJ from oral bisphosphonates has been estimated at 4-8%.** The risk for BRONJ from oral bisphosphonates has been estimated at 4-8%.[15,16] In an attempt to avoid BRONJ, dentists routinely ask patients to discontinue these medications before they'll do an invasive procedure.

Drug manufacturers must include these risks in the package inserts. A drug package insert is an FDA-required document that provides the technical details about drugs for pharmacists and doctors. And while they're not provided to patients, you can easily find them online. Simply Google the name of any medication and "package insert" (eg, search "Fosamax package insert") and you'll find a PDF of the package insert file you can view. For example, if you read the package insert for Prolia, you'll discover that it too can cause osteonecrosis of the jaw.

## Your Level of Commitment

In order to get the benefits, osteoporosis medications must be taken 70-80% of the time.[17] Therefore, you have to be willing to commit to taking it consistently year after year. This is crucial. Because of side effects and how challenging it can be to take some of the medications, 50% of all patients who start osteoporosis meds stop refilling their prescriptions within a year and 60% stop after two years.[18,19]

Some medications you'll need to take daily, weekly, monthly, every six months or annually. For example, if your prescription is for an oral bisphosphonate, you'll need to take it on an empty stomach, daily or once a week, while standing up for at least 30 minutes to prevent damage to your esophagus (the tube from your mouth to your stomach). If you're prescribed the parathyroid hormone medication Forteo, you'll need to give yourself a daily injection under the skin in your thigh or abdomen. And if you take Prolia, it's injected by your healthcare provider once every six months.

Ask your doctor how long you'll be on the medication and what happens after you finish it. Frequently, they'll want you to switch to a different drug. For example, once you finish Forteo, you'll probably be recommended a bisphosphonate. It's important you understand the entire treatment plan and make sure you're comfortable with it.

## 🦴 Take Action 🦴

If you have a doctor's appointment, make sure to have your questions written down in advance. It can be difficult to remember all the questions, so make sure you're prepared. To make it easier, I've included the questions below and in a PDF you can get at nbihealth.com/osteobook. Print it out, answer the questions and take it with you to your appointment.

If you're taking an osteoporosis medication and are now wondering if it's the right choice, call your healthcare provider and make an appointment to discuss it. If you're going to a doctor's appointment to discuss osteoporosis and you're not taking a medication, most likely this topic will come up.

## Questions to ask your doctor:

1. What kind of osteoporosis do I have (eg, post-menopausal osteoporosis, medication-induced osteoporosis)?

_____

2. If my osteoporosis is caused by a medication....

   a. which one? _____

   b. can I lower the dose, discontinue the medication or switch to a safer one? _____

3. Has the osteoporosis medication been shown in clinical trials to prevent fractures in someone with my diagnosis (eg, postmenopausal osteoporosis or medication-induced osteoporosis)?

_____

4. Have you ever had an osteoporosis fracture? ____

   a. If your answer is No, has the medication been shown in clinical trials to work for primary fracture prevention? _____

i. **If No**, ask your doctor why they're recommending the medication.

ii. **If Yes**, which fractures does it prevent (eg, vertebral, hip)? _____

If the medication doesn't prevent both vertebral and hip fractures, ask your doctor what they can recommend to give you greater fracture protection.

b. **If your answer is Yes**, has the medication been shown in clinical trials to work for secondary fracture prevention?

_____

i. **If No**, ask your doctor why they're recommending that specific medication.

ii. **If Yes**, which fractures does it prevent (eg, vertebral, hip)? _____

If the medication doesn't prevent both vertebral and hip fractures, ask your doctor what they can recommend that will give greater fracture protection.

5. How would I take the medication and how frequently (eg, standing up, orally, injection, infusion)?

6. What are the potential side effects and the percentage of people who experience them? (If your doctor doesn't know off the top of their head, ask for the drug package insert. This information is listed in Sections 5 and 6 of the FDA-required package inserts.)

7. How long will you have to take the medication?

8. What's the long-term plan? When you're done taking it, will you stop all osteoporosis medications or be switched to a different one? (If the doctor wants to switch you to a different one, then ask these same questions about the additional medication.)

## Chapter 7

# The Osteoporosis Diet

Most Americans are overfed and malnourished. The typical diet is destroying bones and creating the perfect environment for developing chronic diseases and shaving years off our precious time on Earth. If you eat like the average American you're consuming about 2,100 calories per day and a ton of food—nearly 2,000 pounds—every year.[1,2] If all of it were healthy, nutritious food, that would be fantastic. But it's not. Not even close.

There's only so much food we can eat during the day, so if you're filling up with poor quality foods, that means you're not eating enough of the good stuff. Data collected by the CDC's Behavioral Risk Factors Survey in 2019 revealed that 40% of US adults eat less than one fruit and 22% eat less than one vegetable per day.[3] You know what people are eating a lot of? Refined, sugary, nutrient-deficient food. In 2014 alone, Americans ate 20 billion donuts. That's 63 donuts per person. Love ice cream? Apparently so do a lot of other folks—to the tune of 15 billion pints (47 pints per person) a year.

A review of 49 studies from more than 20 countries showed that the Western dietary pattern is associated with lower bone mineral density and increased osteoporosis and fracture risk.[4] It's because this diet is packed with soft drinks, fried foods, meat, processed foods, sweets, desserts and refined grains. In addition to increasing the risk for nutritional deficiencies and all the damage that creates, the Standard American Diet damages bone by promoting low-grade, chronic inflammation.[5] Unfortunately, this is how most Americans eat, which could explain why there's an epidemic of osteoporosis, heart disease, diabetes, obesity and other diseases that can largely be prevented and improved with diet.

The fact that eating this way causes all these diseases isn't surprising. Processed foods such as white rice, pasta, potato chips and baked goods that use white flour are nearly devoid of vitamins and minerals.[6,7] These foods are consumed in large quantities in the United States and are a cause of nutritional deficiencies. The nutrition that's lost during the process of refining wheat to make white flour for breads, muffins, cookies, and pizza dough is staggering: 85% of magnesium, 60% of calcium, 68% of copper, 76% of iron, 77% of potassium, 78% of zinc, 86% of manganese, 50-80% of all B vitamins and 86% of other vitamins.[8,9] The naturally occurring nutrients are destroyed by removing the most nutrient-dense portion of the grain and applying heat during the manufacturing process. Deficiencies in these and other nutrients create dysfunctions in biochemical pathways that cause chronic inflammation and degenerative conditions like cardiovascular disease and osteoporosis.

In contrast, a healthy diet that's rich in fruits, vegetables, whole grains, nuts, legumes and lean proteins like poultry and fish is associated with increased bone mineral density and lower fracture risk.[10-12] One dietary pattern that has consistently been shown to lower osteoporosis and fracture risk is the Mediterranean Diet. It's how many cultures have traditionally eaten for centuries in that region, including southwestern France, Spain and Italy. In these countries, people following the Mediterranean Diet eat far more whole foods than Americans do. These include foods like fish and other seafood, olive oil, legumes, seeds and nuts, whole grain rice and root vegetables.

There's also a difference in the kinds of fats consumed. Approximately 40% of the energy consumed in the Mediterranean Diet comes from fat, which is relatively high and goes against the "low fat diet" craze popular in the US. But our bodies need fat. Our brains are 60% fat, and fat is needed for mood, a healthy nervous system, hormone production and the immune system. Unlike the Standard American Diet, the Mediterranean Diet emphasizes healthy fats from olive oil, nuts, seeds and fish.[13]

Essentially, following this whole-foods approach provides a long list of both macro- and micronutrients the body uses for bone health. Consuming foods rich in healthy fats and lean proteins, as well as plants rich in magnesium, manganese, potassium, phosphorous, calcium, iron, vitamin K, vitamin B12, folate and vitamins C, D and E is associated with a lower risk of bone fractures.[14] Plus, fruits and vegetables have powerful antioxidants called polyphenols and gut-healthy fiber.

The more someone sticks to eating this way the better. One study that evaluated the dietary patterns of more than 70,000 women and men concluded that the more someone adhered to a Mediterranean dietary pattern the greater the health bene-fits.[15] Compared to those who only loosely followed this way of eating, people who most strictly ate this way had an incred-ible 22% decrease in total fracture risk from diet alone.

Supporting these findings, researchers looked at dietary patterns of postmenopausal women and found that those who more closely followed a Mediterranean Diet had a 20% decreased risk of hip fractures.[16] Hip frac-tures are the most dan-gerous type of osteo-porosis fracture. If you have osteoporosis and break a hip, your risk for dying is increased for up to 10 years after. Reducing hip fracture risk by 20% simply by changing how you eat is a no-brainer.[17]

> Researchers looked at dietary patterns of postmenopausal women and found that those who more closely followed a Mediterranean Diet had an incredible 20% decreased risk of hip fractures.

One reason why this diet is so healthy is because fruits and vegetables have high amounts of dietary nitrates. Nitrates found naturally in plants improve blood flow and are associat-ed with increased muscle function and strength in elderly men and women.[18,19] Foods with the highest amounts of nitrates are green leafy vegetables such as spinach, beet leaves, lettuce and parsley. Beet roots are also an excellent source. But don't worry about tracking how much nitrates or other nutrients you're getting. The beauty of eating a predominantly whole-foods diet with lots of different vegetables and fruits is that it provides a wealth of protective nutrients.

Since you have to eat, you might as well be doing something good for yourself instead of increasing your risk for a future of pain, disability and an early death. The science is clear. It's in your best interest to eat a whole-foods, Mediterranean Diet. This way of eating is not a fad diet. It's a lifestyle. And despite its name, it's not a diet in the traditional sense. One of the problems with diets is that they tend to be restrictive. They focus on what you shouldn't eat instead of teaching you how to eat and helping you transition into eating that way.

I've adopted the Mediterranean Diet to specifically focus on emphasizing an approach that builds stronger bones and called it the Osteoporosis Diet. It's a way of feeding your body nutritious, wholesome food that reduces your osteoporosis and fracture risk. It can also increase muscle mass, which makes you stronger, improves your balance and decreases your risk for falling. Eating healthy, however, doesn't only help your bones and muscles. This dietary pattern also reduces your risk for heart disease, dementia, strokes, diabetes, obesity and cancer and gives you more energy, improves your mood and helps you feel and look your best.

It's not a diet where I tell you what you need to avoid. Instead, my Osteoporosis Diet teaches you how you should eat most of the time to promote your health for the rest of your life. Over many years in my medical practice helping people transition into eating this way, I distilled the healthy diet recommendations into a simple three-step system. And within that, you only need to focus on two food groups: plants and protein.

## Plants

Plants provide fiber, vitamins, minerals and other plant nutrients your body needs to thrive. Green leafy vegetables like lettuce, chard and kale contain lots of magnesium, potassium and vitamin K. Colorful vegetables like bell peppers and carrots contain powerful plant carotenoids and other plant antioxidants. Eating a rainbow a day of different colored fruits and vegetables gives you a variety of nutrients your body needs.

Fiber is one of those important nutrients. Fiber helps you feel full longer. It helps regulates blood sugar. And it's important for healthy gut bacteria. In the large intestines, fiber increases the production of an important short chain fatty acid called butyrate. Butyrate has lots of health benefits, including promoting bone health.[20]

Unfortunately, most people don't eat enough fiber, which means they're not eating enough plants. In 2018, Americans only consumed an average of 16 grams of dietary fiber per day.[21] That's about half of what people should be eating and about ten times less than our ancestral diets. It's been estimated that when humans were hunter-gatherers, we consumed about 150 grams of fiber per day.[22]

> Most people don't eat enough fiber, which means they're not eating enough plants.

I want people to eat a minimum of 30 grams of dietary fiber a day. If you're eating 30 grams of dietary fiber every day, you'll naturally be eating lots of whole foods. But it's not only the fiber that's important. It's where the fiber is found. Dietary fiber is in whole fruits and vegetables. And the best way to understand if you're getting enough is to track how much fiber you're eating.

This is easy to calculate, and below I'll walk you through exactly how to do that and how to develop an intuitive sense of how to eat healthy. Eating optimally will become a habit and not a struggle. But eating enough plants to get enough fiber is only half of the puzzle. You also need lots of healthy protein.

## Protein

Proteins contain amino acids, which combine to form more than 500,000 different proteins in the body for hormones, muscle, tendons, bone, your immune system and much more. There are more than 250 proteins in bones alone, so you can't have healthy bones (or a healthy body) without protein.

Despite the keto, high-protein craze, too many people aren't consuming the recommended daily amount (RDA) of protein. According to the research, 38% of adult men and 41% of adult women eat less than the RDA, and 15% of people older than 60 years consume less than 75%.[23,24]

When you don't get enough protein, you lose bone and muscle. Muscle loss is so common as we age that it's estimated that people lose about 3-5% of their muscle per year, so that an 80-year-old person will have 15-25% less skeletal muscle than they did when they were younger.[25] When that happens,

**When you don't get enough protein, you lose bone and muscle.**

strength and balance decrease and falls and fracture risks go up. People with both osteoporosis and muscle loss have a condition called osteosarcopenia. Men with osteosarcopenia have a 349% increased risk for fractures compared to men with healthy bone and muscle mass.[26] When a man with this condition gets a hip fracture, his risk for dying within one year is 26% higher than a man without osteosarcopenia.[27]

Surprisingly, osteosarcopenia in women doesn't appear to increase their risk for dying. It's a mystery why, but it might be because diseases in older men tend to be more severe than in older women. This puts men at greater risk for the deadly effects of an osteoporotic hip fracture. In fact, men with osteoporosis who break a hip are up to twice as likely to die compared to women.[28]

To build stronger bones and muscles, the research suggests a minimum protein intake of 1.0 to 1.3 grams per kilogram (g/kg) body weight per day, plus resistance training.[29] And other recommendations go as high as 2.0 g/kg body weight per day.[23] I'll help you with the resistance training and exercise part in the next chapter, but just eating enough protein can protect your bones. In a study of women ages 65-72, those who ate more than 1.2 grams of protein per kilogram body weight per day and who also supplemented with calcium and vitamin D for three years, had significantly higher bone mineral density compared to those who ate less protein.[30]

I know a lot of people don't love math, but stick with me, because you need to learn to calculate how much protein you should be eating for your body weight. It's actually quite easy and only involves two steps. So grab a calculator. Unless your doctor has put you on a low-protein diet for some reason (eg, you have kidney failure), I recommend shooting for at least 1.3 g of protein per kilogram body weight per day. Here's a simple way to determine how many grams to eat.

1. Convert your body weight from pounds to kilograms. To do this, take your body weight in pounds and divide it by 2.2.

**I weigh: _____ kilograms.**

2. Next, take your weight in kilograms and multiply it by 1.3. The result is the minimum number of grams of protein you need to eat each day. Round up or down to the nearest whole number to make it easier.

**I will eat: _____ grams of protein per day.**

Here's a real-life example. I weigh 150 pounds, so let's figure out how many grams of protein I should be eating every day.

1. 150 lbs ÷ 2.2 kg/lb = 68 kg

2. 68 kg x 1.3 g/kg = 88.4 grams of protein. For simplicity, I'd simply round up and say I should be eating at least 89 grams of protein per day.

## Know Your Numbers

I have yet to meet anyone who could tell me how much dietary fiber is in an apple, lettuce or a pear. Or how much protein is in the different foods they're eating. To transition into this way of eating, you'll need to quantify how many grams of fiber and protein you're eating. It's actually quite simple.

If you're eating pre-packaged foods, the nutrition facts panel will tell you how many grams of fiber and protein there are in a serving. You can then estimate how many servings you're eating and how many grams of fiber and protein you're getting.

For whole, unpackaged foods like celery or a serving of chicken, there aren't handy nutrition facts panels to glance at. To help you, I created handouts of fiber and protein content for commonly consumed foods. They're included in the Appendix. You can also print them out from nbihealth.com/osteobook and use them as references. And if what you're looking for isn't on those handouts, a quick Google search can fill in the gaps.

## ♫ Take Action ♫

Below I walk you through the steps to transition into eating this way.

### Step 1. Calculate Where You're At

If you're excited to start increasing your protein and fiber, I'm thrilled. But first I want you to figure out how much protein and fiber you're currently eating so you have proof of the changes you need to make.

Use the handy Plants and Protein tables in the Appendix. Take a piece of paper, keep a Note on your phone or download and use one of the many food tracking apps. Log everything you eat for two days.

At the end of each day, estimate how many grams of total fiber and protein you ate. An easy way to do this is to find the food on the Plants and Protein tables at the end of this book. If it's a packaged food, look on the Nutrition Facts Panel and estimate the amount from there. Make sure to take into account the serving size.

For example, on the Nutrition Facts panel of a can of kidney beans, the serving size is half a cup. Each serving provides 7 grams of protein and 8 grams of dietary fiber. If I eat half a cup of kidney beans, I'll log those amounts in my tracker.

When you've completed your two days of track-ing, you'll have your baseline and know what to increase and by how much.

**Step 2. Transition into Eating This Way**

After you've calculated your baseline (how many grams of proteins and fiber you're eating before you changed your diet) you can start transitioning into your new eating lifestyle. Most of the time people find that eating more of a whole foods diet—with more fruits, vegetables and protein—is a big change and it can take some time to transition. It might require shopping differently (including doing most of your shopping in the outermost aisles of the store), cooking differently and perhaps using dif-ferent herbs and spices. Check your mindset and approach it as a fun way to explore new flavors, feel more vibrant and look better.

I like to tell people to transition over six weeks because major changes done overnight tend to be unsustainable long-term. People like to have some-thing to look forward to, especially during the tran-sition. So try following this for six days a week, and on the seventh day eat whatever you want. What you'll discover is that you're feeling healthier and getting leaner, but on the seventh day when you go off the diet and are eating like crap, you'll feel like crap too.

You'll also notice that your taste buds will change. Since you'll be eating less refined sugar, you'll taste more of the natural sweetness in fruits and some vegetables. Your taste buds and your body will adapt to this way of eating, and you'll start to crave healthy, nutritious foods that your body thrives on.

**Step 3. Develop a New Habit**

As you're developing your new eating habit, rely on the Plants and Protein tables in the Appendix and be diligent about calculating the amounts you're getting. But only for a little while. The tables are tools to help you do that. I don't want you to have to rely on handouts the rest of your life. The goal is to develop an intuitive sense of what it means to eat healthy so that as you're cooking or looking down at your plate, you just know when you're doing it right. Once you understand how to eat like this, you can simply stick the handouts in a drawer, or better yet share them with a friend and help them too.

## Chapter 8

# Too Fit to Fracture

Decreasing your fracture risk with exercise requires you focus on two things: balance and strength. Ninety-five percent of all fractures happen because someone falls. So it's simple—if you prevent yourself from falling, you'll prevent yourself from breaking a bone, hitting your head, or having a nasty bruise or any of the other problems caused by taking a spill.

**Ninety-five percent of all fractures happen because someone falls.**

It's important to recognize that there isn't a one-size-fits-all recommendation. Lifting weights or doing sit-ups may be safe in someone with mild osteoporosis, but dangerous for people with severe osteoporosis. To find the right exercise for you, you must carefully evaluate and define the type, intensity, and duration of a program that will be safe. Some yoga or Pilates exercises may be fantastic for improving balance and strength in someone with osteoporosis. Yet without modifications and an instructor trained as an osteoporosis exercise specialist, even gentle yoga or Pilates may cause fractures in people with osteoporosis where the bones are already quite fragile.

For example, flexion exercises—where you bend forward—like sit-ups and crunches puts a lot of stress on the front of your spine and can cause fractures. Add in kyphosis and you've at even more risk. Kyphosis, also called Dowager's hump, is a head-forward posture with a hump in the upper back that puts an abnormal amount of pressure on the front of the spine. When these fractures occur, they're called *compression fractures* because the added pressure on your spine is what breaks the bones.

A study in 1984 evaluated different types of exercises in 59 volunteers with postmenopausal osteoporosis. Even though doctors recommended exercise at the time for osteoporosis, this was the first study to evaluate the effects that specific types of exercises—flexion, extension or a combination of the two—have on fracture risk. Women were prescribed exercises, such as back extensions while lying down (Picture 1), extension in a seated position (Picture 2), stretching the back muscles by bending forward while sitting in a chair (Picture 3) and sit ups (Picture 4). After about one and a half to two years, 16% of women doing the extension exercises had new spine fractures while 89% of those doing flexion exercises and 53% of those doing a combination of flexion and extension exercises had new spinal fractures.[1]

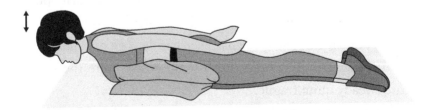

**Picture 1.**
Back extension exercise while lying down.

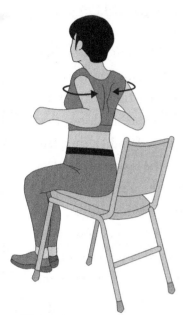

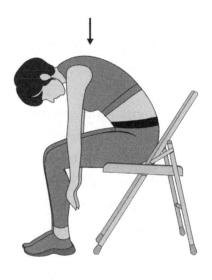

**Picture 2.**
Seated back extension exercise.

**Picture 3.**
Stretching the back muscle while seated in a chair bending forward.

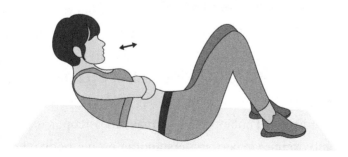

**Picture 4.**
Sit-ups increase abdominal muscle strength but put extra stress on the front of the spine.

Rapid twisting, like what happens during a golf swing, can also cause a fracture. Certain yoga poses like pigeon that put high amounts of stress on the pelvis, could result in a broken hip. Compression fractures can also occur during inverted poses and pulling your knees to your chest in a tight ball. Even riding your bike can injure your spine. These are all things that many at-risk people do daily because they're familiar, they feel good, and no one has ever taught them the risks involved or evaluated the activities to make sure they're safe.

This isn't meant to scare you into inaction. Quite the opposite. Exercising is crucially important to your bones and overall health. The challenge is that most people were never taught how to exercise properly, and many instructors aren't trained how to work with people with osteoporosis. How we exercise as we age, especially with osteoporosis, should not be the same as how you did it in your twenties or thirties. Your body has changed, and if you don't adapt with it, instead of decreasing your risk of a fracture, you'll be increasing it.

**Your body has changed, and if you don't adapt with it, instead of decreasing your risk of a fracture, you'll be increasing it.**

According to Penelope Wasserman, an osteoporosis movement and exercise expert, understanding proper body mechanics and how to move without putting yourself at risk is crucial. She served on the Eli Lilly Mobility Advisory Board, founded Million Dollar Bones and created the Internal Alignment

Awareness training program to teach healthy, safe alignment techniques to prevent osteoporosis related fractures. Penelope advocates finding an excellent program and instructor to help you learn how to exercise in a way that's safe and effective. Doing so will also help improve how you move during routine activities throughout the day—sitting, walking, bending over to pick something up, twisting to look behind you and emptying the dishwasher. During the interview with her for my Delivering Health podcast, I asked Penelope how people with osteoporosis can exercise safely. She said, "Awareness of proper spinal and hip alignment should be part of any approach. Learning how your bones support you in space and developing an awareness of how your body moves will give you the foundation you need to choose the safest and smartest exercise routine for your body."

Deciding what's appropriate for you is based on your muscle strength, range of motion, balance, gait, heart and lung health, additional diseases you may have, bone density, whether you have a history of previous fractures and an assessment of your fall risk. I know as I've gotten older, even though my mind thinks I'm still in my 20s, my body lets me know I'm not. For years while I was in medical school, starting my clinic, having our two children, growing my dietary supplement company and writing books, I got out of shape. When I decided to start exercising again, however, I jumped right back into lifting weights and running at the same intensity as I did 15 years earlier. I kept getting injured until I worked with a trainer who could help me slowly and carefully get back in shape.

To create a safe and effective program, an exercise professional needs to understand your goals and your current condition. They also must evaluate how you walk, whether you have a history of falls or surgery, and how you use your body throughout the day. For example, do you sit all day or stand for long stretches of time? You should identify anything that can change your risk before you start working out. Failure to do so can create abnormal and dangerous stresses on your body.

It's dangerous to assume a Pilates or yoga instructor or a personal trainer understands how to work with someone with osteoporosis. Before you sign on with anyone, it's important to interview them. Penelope recommends asking the following questions:

- Are you familiar with osteoporosis?
- Do you have training in working with people who have osteoporosis?
- Do you know which exercises to avoid in an osteoporosis exercise program?
- Do you have other clients with osteoporosis?

The most intense exercises, such as high-impact activities, that are effective in increasing bone mass in young people may not be appropriate for some older people with osteoporosis.

That said, there's almost always something people can do to improve their balance and strength.

And almost anyone can do the Stork Exercise. It's one of my favorites because it's a simple exercise you can do to improve your balance and reduce your risk of falling and fall-related injuries. Storks are famous for standing on one leg. That's what you're going to do every time you brush your teeth. While you're spending one minute on the bottom teeth, stand on one leg. Feel the floor with your foot and imagine the ground reaction force lifting through your arch to help keep you upright and balanced as you lift one foot to stand like a stork. You can grab the counter to steady yourself if you need it, but work over time to let go.

When you move to the top teeth, spend another minute standing on the other leg. Again, steady yourself as needed. And that's your two minutes, twice a day. For two minutes, twice a day, be a stork.

If you have an electric toothbrush, like a Sonicare or something similar, it keeps track of the two minutes for you. Many electric toothbrushes beep to let you know when it's time to switch to the top teeth and are programmed to turn off automatically when time's up. If your toothbrush isn't as fancy, set the timer on your phone.

Once you master the Stork Exercise, start brushing your teeth with your opposite hand to create a new challenge for your brain and your balance.

The Stork Exercise tightens your core a little bit, engages your supporting muscles in your legs, improves your balance and can reduce the risk of falling. I've been teaching patients this simple and powerful exercise for years. To get the most out of it—like with any exercise—you need to do it consistently. Try it twice a day for a few weeks. You'll feel steadier, stronger and more confident knowing that you're taking a powerful step toward reducing your fracture risk.

As I talk about later in the chapter, daily physical activity that you normally do around the house can also be turned into bone-healthy activities. But before I go into that and provide recommendations for more balance and strength exercises, let's look at how Americans overall are doing in the exercise department.

Even though everyone knows they should exercise, too many aren't. The average adult spends more than half of their waking hours sitting around. Sitting at work, watching television at home, playing video games, riding in a car. If tapping the keyboard at a desk job or scrolling through funny videos and pictures of cute animals on Facebook were considered exercise, we'd all be in phenomenal shape.

Even children are sitting around a lot more these days, which doesn't bode well for their health or their bones as they get older. An estimated 29% of all Americans over the age of six years old are inactive, meaning they don't engage in any regular physical activity. Unfortunately, as people get older, they move their butts even less. More than 40% of people 65 years old or older aren't doing *any* regular physical activity.[2]

A hundred years ago, sitting jobs were almost unheard of, walking was common and obesity wasn't a public health crisis.

People worked more in factories or jobs that required them to stand and move all day. Now there are screens seemingly everywhere to occupy peoples' time. Sitting around may seem like a normal way of life these days, but just because everyone else seems to be doing it doesn't make it good for you—or them. Studies consistently show that the more sedentary you are, the greater your risk for getting many chronic diseases, including diabetes, breast cancer and osteoporosis.[3-5] A sedentary life is also bad for your mood and increases your risk for depression by 25% compared to folks who regularly exercise.[6]

> Studies consistently show that the more sedentary you are, the greater your risk for getting many chronic diseases, including diabetes, breast cancer and osteoporosis.

Not only does being a couch potato make you sick, it makes what you've already got worse. People with arthritis who don't participate in regular exercise have more severe pain and decreased physical function.[7] If your memory or ability to process information is declining, being sedentary worsens cognitive function in older adults.[8]

And if all that weren't enough to get you moving consistently, being sedentary doesn't only increase your risk of diseases and can make those you have worse, it can kill you. A 2014 review of studies reported that being sedentary for more than eight hours a day increases the risk of death from any cause, and the longer you sit around, the greater your risk.[9] One study found that women who sat for 11 or more hours a day had a

52% higher risk of death than women who sat for less than eight hours per day.[10] A 2015 meta-analysis found that not exercising increases your risk of dying from heart disease and cancer by nearly 20%.[11]

The beautiful thing about moving more is that it can improve all areas of your health—cardiovascular, emotional, mental, musculoskeletal—and reduce your risk for dying. That includes reducing your risk from dying from a hip fracture. Moderate physical activity is associated with decreasing hip fracture risk by 45%.[12] That's better than bisphosphonates like alendronate (Fosamax) and Zometa. And all you have to do is get off your keister and move.

> Moderate physical activity is associated with decreasing hip fracture risk by 45%. That's better than bisphosphonates.

There's a lot of confusion out there about what counts as moderate or vigorous exercise. The simplest way to understand it is with the "Talk Test." Moderate exercise means you're moving your body enough so that you're a bit winded but can still carry on a conversation; however, you won't be able to sing. Similarly, you know you're doing vigorous exercise if you're so winded you can't carry on a conversation.

But move how? And how much? There's a common misconception that a person needs to pump iron at the gym or run for miles at a time to achieve the full benefits of exercise. And that's why a lot of people don't ever start or get bored or overwhelmed and quit. But this simply isn't true.

A 2015 article published in the Journal of the American

Medical Association (JAMA), concluded that it only takes 15 minutes per day of moderate exercise for people to start experiencing health benefits.[13] People who did this lost weight, saw improvements in their blood pressure and blood sugar control and reduced their risk for cancer and death. Similar results can be achieved with just 5-10 minutes per day of vigorous exercise such as jogging.

While 15 minutes a day of moderate exercise can improve your health, if you want to exercise longer, you can get even greater improvement. Health benefits of exercise increase with longer duration or intensity until about 90 minutes per day, then plateaus beyond that.

## The 10,000 Steps Myth

One of the beautiful things about exercise is that it can accommodate nearly anyone's preference. If you'd rather track your steps than how long you exercise, you can. For many years I've heard and read on the internet recommendations that people should take 10,000 steps a day. It's always been stated as an indisputable fact. When I hear people make a statement about the health effects of doing something, the doctor and scientist in me thinks, "show me the data." I never thought it was a bad recommendation. I just wasn't sure it was true.

When I heard about the 10,000 step per day rule, I did what I often do—I looked for the research. At that time, and this was several years ago, there weren't any studies that had evaluated the number of steps people took every day. Despite the lack of research, somehow people believed 10,000 steps per day was a proven fact.

Three recent studies tested this assumption. In a clinical trial published in 2021, researchers looked at the risk for death in more than 2,110 volunteers they followed for nearly 11 years. During that time, they tracked the number of steps they took and how vigorously they walked (the intensity). What they found was that people who took an average of 7,000-10,000 steps per day had a 50-70% decreased risk for dying from any cause compared to those who took less than 7,000 steps per day. Taking more than 10,000 steps was not associated with greater benefits.[14] Another study showed again that more isn't necessarily better. They confirmed that taking around 7,000 steps per day is associated with decreased risk for dying, but there wasn't any increased benefit for people taking 12,000 steps.[15]

But 7,000-10,000 steps is a big range. Is there an ideal number of steps that gives the greatest benefit? Fortunately for us, another set of researchers asked this question and discovered that the health benefit plateaued at 7,500 steps per day.[16]

For me these studies were a breath of fresh air. While the 10,000-step goal always felt a bit overwhelming, 7,000-7,500 steps a day is certainly something I can do. So how far is 7,000 steps? People take about 2,000 steps to walk a mile, so 7,000 steps would be about 3.5 miles a day.

The beautiful thing is that all the steps you take during the day count. While you can carve out a specific block of time to get them in, you don't have to. Add steps to your day by parking farther from the entrances of stores, take the stairs instead of the elevator or escalator, pace or walk around the block while you're on the phone or take your dog for a walk. And if you want to know how you're doing, use a step tracker app on your smartphone or buy a separate fitness tracker and get those 7,000 steps in a day.

## Weights or No Weights?

Weight-bearing exercises can promote bone growth and improve balance. Non-weight-bearing exercises can improve your strength and balance. I recommend doing a mix of the two types of exercises. Which exercises you do is only limited by your imagination and an evaluation of what is safe and appropriate. Examples of moderate exercise include brisk walking, bicycling (at a pace slower than 10 miles per hour), water aerobics, ballroom dancing, general gardening or housework. If cycling is your thing, you may want to consider riding a recumbent bike since it puts less pressure on the spine and hips than a standard upright bike. Examples of vigorous exercise include jogging, running, swimming laps, aerobic dancing, jumping rope, or hiking up a mountain with a heavy backpack. Using exercise poles for walking and hiking will improve core strength and balance.

## Exercise Mindset

A positive mindset about exercise can even lead to a cleaner house. If you consider housework as beneficial and as exercise, it can produce some great results. A 2007 study evaluated the effect of mindset on the health of hotel cleaning staff.[17] Some in the group of 84 women were told cleaning was good exercise and informed about the health benefits.

During the following month they were reminded of the health benefits. After four weeks, those who had been told that their work actually *was* exercise believed they were exercising more than before. But the effects weren't all in their heads. Their weight, blood pressure, body fat and waist-to-hip ratio all decreased.

This study shows the importance of intention. While setting aside time for exercise is important, don't forget that what you do normally during the day can also count. When I read this study, a lightbulb went on. I do something around the house every day, and I'm sure you do too.

> While setting aside time for exercise is important, don't forget what you do normally during the day can also count.

Whether it's unloading the dishwasher, reaching up to grab a glass, bending down to get a plate out of a cupboard or typing at my computer, I now intentionally see this as an opportunity to get stronger.

For example, when you reach for a glass, try standing slightly further away to stretch your back muscles. Maybe move a little slower when you do it, and hold your arm out fully extended a little longer to get an even better stretch. And when I vacuum, I switch between my dominant and non-dominant arms so I'm giving them more equal work.

Ultimately, it's all about working your body so your body works for you. To get started, change the way you think about exercise. You don't have to go to the gym or carve large chunks of time out of your day. Between exercise apps, videos and the things you already have in your house (stairs, floor space to do squats and jogging in place), your office (stairs, the block around your building) and your neighborhood (speed walking hills around in your neighborhood), you'll easily get in 20 minutes of movement a day. Most people probably waste more than 20 minutes every day scrolling mindlessly on social media. So instead, put on a podcast, an audiobook or some good music and move.

## Mix It Up

I suggest mixing things up so you're not doing the same thing two days in a row. Variety is the spice of life! And that goes for exercise too. When you're moving your body, you'll not only be doing something positive to reduce your fracture risk, but you'll also feel better. When you take these actions you'll release more of your body's happy chemicals, like dopamine and serotonin. So get out there, move your butt and have some fun.

There's so much you can do and explore. You can go for a walk. One study that reviewed data from nearly half a million healthy people, looked at the effect regular walking has on the risk of developing cardiovascular disease. The study found that the people who walked the most experienced a 31% lower risk of developing cardiovascular disease and a 32% lower risk of dying than people who walked the least.[18] And the more the person walked, the greater the benefit.

If strength training or working your flexibility or balance is more your thing, then pursue activities that help you work on improving those areas of your health. A study comparing the effects of aerobic exercise with yoga and tai chi found that all three types of exercise provide equal physical benefits, but only the yoga and tai chi also improved mood and sleep.[19] A published case study showed that salsa dancing can benefit patients with Alzheimer's disease.[20] Salsa dancing can also be a great aerobic workout that can improve your balance.

There are so many other activities to explore: swimming, gardening, modified Pilates, modified Yoga, paddle boarding or practicing Qi gong. The opportunities to move your body and improve your health are endless. Get creative and have fun. You can take classes or enlist an exercise buddy or group of friends to help you stay motivated. The point is that participating in physical activity on a regular basis will get you on the path to being too fit to fracture while also feeling and looking better, and who doesn't want that?

### Schedule Your Exercise

Put it on the calendar and make non-negotiable appointments with yourself to exercise. This is easy if it's a class, but people don't do this for solo activities like going for a walk or doing yoga at home. No wonder it often doesn't happen. Treat it like a business appointment and commit to following through.

## ♪ Take Action ♪

Answer these questions to help you get organized and get started. You can also download them from nbihealth.com/osteobook.

**Write down as many activities you can think of that you love:**

_____

_____

_____

**Which activities can you do by yourself?**

_____

_____

_____

_____

**Which require a class?**

_____

_____

_____

_____

If any of your activities are done in a class, write down the name of the studio and the class. If you don't know a place that offers what you need, find it now.

_____

_____

_____

Which activities do you want to do with a friend? Write them down, along with the friend's name.

_____

_____

_____

_____

_____

If you want to exercise with friends or your partner, call or text them now. Seriously. Stop reading and reach out to them now. Then add your exercise to your calendar for the next week so you know exactly what, when and where you'll exercise.

## Chapter 9

# Find Your Zen

M ost of us are under a bone-killing amount of stress. A global pandemic upended our lives. Political and social divisions are constantly highlighted in the news and social media. And we've been led to believe that without pain we haven't accomplished or achieved.

The chronic stress takes its toll. According to the American Psychological Association (APA), 75% of Americans experience symptoms of stress, including lying awake at night, feeling nervous or anxious, irritability or anger and fatigue."[1] And that was before the pandemic. Since then, it's only gotten worse. So much so that APA's Stress in America survey for 2020 concluded that the pandemic has created "a national mental health crisis that could yield serious health and social consequences for years to come."[2]

Since one of my obsessions is the fight against osteoporosis, I of course want to understand how this increased stress can cause or exacerbate the disease and increase fracture risk.

The body has amazing ways for adapting to its environment. For many people under chronic stress, they may in fact just think it's normal. But just because people perceive it as the norm, doesn't make it acceptable. Even though we can get used to living with stress and the high levels of stress hormones that come with it, that doesn't mean we should. The havoc it causes on our health should be a wake-up call to anyone reading this.

Chronic stress activates your hypothalamic-pituitary-adrenal (HPA) axis and the sympathetic nervous system (SNS), which regulate your response to challenges and threats. This includes anxiety about current events, fighting off the common cold, worrying about finances, feeling overwhelmed with work and the stories you tell yourself about what might happen in the future.

Your HPA axis is composed of two small areas in the brain called the hypothalamus and the pituitary gland. These are connected by nerves to your adrenal glands, which sit on top of your kidneys. To rally the body's resources to handle stress, your brain sends signals to the adrenal glands to release stress hormones such as epinephrine, norepinephrine and cortisol. In the process, however, dangerous free radicals are created.

Over the short term, the stress response is adaptive. It helps us handle things better, enhances immune function and helps us focus. But long-term stress has the opposite effects. It's linked to lowered immune function, elevated blood pressure, and increased heart rate.[3] Chronic stress also contributes to insomnia, heart disease, dementia, leaky gut, dysbiosis, osteoporosis, sagging skin and arthritis. And it shrinks your brain.[4-6]

We've known for decades that high cortisol levels create osteoporosis. As I discussed in Chapter 5, medications that artificially elevate cortisol like prednisone and dexamethasone increase osteoporosis and fracture risk up to 200%. But your body's own production of cortisol can destroy bone too.

Cushing's disease is a medical condition in which the adrenal glands produce too much cortisol and is a secondary cause of osteoporosis. Someone with this disease could have cortisol levels four to five times higher than normal. But studies have shown that even in "normal, healthy" men and women, having cortisol that is toward the higher end of normal is a risk for losing bone faster.[7,8]

Chronic stress strips calcium from bone and increases fracture risk by destroying collagen. Collagen is the most plentiful protein in your body, and it's the key molecule that makes up connective tissue. Collagen is secreted by cells and assembles in networks of thick, rope-like structures called fibrils. Collagen is made up of three strands of repeating amino acids wrapped around each other that create the shape and support for tissues and provides a scaffolding for cell growth and movement.[9] Think about collagen like rebar used in construction, holding everything up.

**Chronic stress strips calcium from bone and increases fracture risk by destroying collagen.**

Collagen is found in your bones, muscles, tendons, ligaments, skin, blood vessels, teeth and in the cornea and vitreous (the gelatinous substance) of your eyes.[10] It provides all these tissues with structure, strength, and flexibility and is critical for the health of all these tissues.[11] Collagen not only makes bone slightly flexible and more able to withstand the impact of a fall without breaking, but it's also the framework to which calcium and other minerals bind. When collagen is destroyed, bones become weaker and more brittle.

Collagen not only makes bone slightly flexible and more able to withstand the impact of a fall without breaking, but it's also the framework to which calcium and other minerals bind.

Chronic stress damages collagen by increasing pro-inflammatory molecules, such as interleukin-1 beta (IL1-beta) and tumor necrosis factor-alpha (TNF-alpha). Over the long term, this can create an imbalance between pro-inflammatory and anti-inflammatory molecules.[12] Like cortisol, chronic elevation of inflammatory molecules damages collagen and reduces your body's ability to make new collagen. [13,14]

If all that weren't enough, inflammation also makes collagen stiffer and less flexible by creating advanced glycation end-products (AGEs) that bind to collagen and damage it. The accumulation of AGEs is associated with poorer vision due to the lens in your eye becoming more rigid, hardening of the arteries, thinner and more fragile skin and tendons and weaker bones.[15,16]

When it comes to osteoporosis, you want to create an environment for your body to grow stronger bones, and in so doing, reduce bone loss and fracture risk. So managing stress is an important part of any holistic approach.

Fortunately, there are simple things you can do now to reduce your stress, reduce your risk and help you start feeling better quickly. Here are my top recommendations. Of course, there are others not listed here that are effective, and I encourage you to explore and find what works best for you. The more you do, the better you'll feel. However, even focusing on just one, two or three will make a world of difference and get your life moving in the direction of a less stressful you.

## Catch Some ZZZs

Sleep deprivation puts a tremendous stress on your body, decreases your ability to think clearly and complete daily tasks and increases cortisol. Make sure you're getting an average of 7.5 to 8 hours of sleep per night. In Chapter 10, I take a deep dive into the reasons why people aren't sleeping well and provide recommendations for how you can improve yours.

## Chill Out

Practicing regular stress reduction techniques is important. It doesn't have to be the same thing every day, but doing something for YOU every day should be non-negotiable. You're worth it and you deserve it. Yoga, meditation, walks, getting out into nature, gardening, prayer and reading for enjoyment can all help. It really doesn't matter what you do, as long as you're consistent. And don't think you have to limit yourself to just one.

What I've found works for me is to typically wake up 45 minutes before everyone else in my family. This is my quiet time before the rest of the house gets up and the day gets crazy. During my "me time" I get my cup of coffee, my journal and my book. I set a timer and read (for pleasure) for 30 minutes, and then take some time to write in my journal or quietly think and set my intentions for the day. Since I know I can't do everything and getting an average of 7.5 hours of sleep a night for me is non-negotiable, this means I'm usually the first one in my family to go to sleep. But it's worth it, because this routine allows me to have more energy, feel more centered and healthier and be more present in their lives and mine.

Also, throughout the week, my wife Romi and I will walk the dog together, my daughter and I will have an occasional coffee date and my son and I may watch a soccer game together. I also make sure to regularly connect with friends and volunteer in my community. All these things give me purpose and fill my "chill out" bucket. They help me feel more connected to myself and others and reduce my stress. Like with anything, find out what works best for you and consistently make it part of your week.

## Nourish Your Body

Poor diet creates chronic inflammation and increases cortisol. When you're not giving your body the raw materials it needs, it can't give you what you need to feel your best. Eat a stress-reducing diet, like my Osteoporosis Diet I discuss in Chapter

10, and make sure to drink plenty of water during the day to stay hydrated.

## Deal with Problems

One of the biggest reasons people feel stressed is because they don't deal with issues that are bothering them. Avoiding the problem doesn't make it go away. In fact, letting problems fester often makes them worse. Facing issues head on, recognizing them, being honest with yourself and others about them, getting the help you need and coming up with a plan to deal with them will help you feel more in control of your life and reduce your stress. After all, we get what we tolerate. If you tolerate feeling less than fantastic, that's what you'll have. If you tolerate people treating you in ways you don't like, that's what

> One of the biggest reasons people feel stressed is because they don't deal with issues that are bothering them. Avoiding the problem doesn't make it go away.

you'll get. And if getting counseling, doing Reiki or any other personal development approach resonates with you, do them. They can all help you get a healthier handle on your life.

## Control Technology

Smartphones and tablets have revolutionized modern life. Although I grew up before these devices were around, I can't imagine life now without them. But for all they've done to improve our lives, being connected 24/7 has no-doubt increased people's stress.

It's important to put limits on your technology. What I've found that works for me is that I spend the first working hour each morning clearing out my inbox. Then I don't check email for most of the rest of the day. I also limit my social media to chunks that are scheduled so I'm not aimlessly scrolling and wasting my time. And since staring at a screen before bed wreaks havoc on sleep, I put my screen down at least an hour before I go to sleep.

## Stop Multitasking

Research shows that multitasking increases stress and makes us less efficient. Multitasking is a myth. Our brains can't simultaneously focus on two tasks at once. Instead, we switch between tasks, a phenomenon called "task switching." Every time we switch tasks, we release a dose of the stress hormone cortisol. It also releases the reward-seeking hormone dopamine and moves the brain's focus away from the thoughtful, reasoned prefrontal cortex to the emotional limbic system.

Instead of multitasking, a popular workflow strategy is to chunk or block tasks during the day. I've been doing this for years now and it's made a world of difference. I'm more productive and more relaxed. Here's how it works: you block out chunks of time to focus on specific tasks, and you don't switch between them. When the time is up, you move to the next task you scheduled. In this way, I can get through all my emails, sit down and plan marketing strategy, work on new product development, record my podcast and handle kid and family stuff. Each one of those is a chunk of time dedicated to that task. Just think how much more relaxed and productive you'd be if you structured more of your weeks like this.

## Get Into Nature

In Japan there's a practice called Shinrin-yoku ("forest bathing" or "nature treatment") in which people immerse themselves in nature like taking a walk in the woods or a garden. Studies on forest bathing show that it improves mood, decreases pain, helps people feel calmer, strengthens the immune system and reduces cortisol and blood pressure.[17] Get into nature and help your body heal.

## Create Your Stop-Doing List

The reason most people are frazzled is because they have a hard time prioritizing themselves, saying no to things that don't serve them and are perpetually overwhelmed and over-committed. Romi once taught me that our stop-doing list is in many ways even more important than our to-do lists. While she was building her now global skincare business, being mom to our two kids and juggling life's other demands, she created and assembled tools to help her recalibrate her life. Since then, she's taught tens of thousands how to do it too, including figuring out what to put on your Stop-Doing List. In her book, *You Can Have it All, Just Not at the Same Damn Time*, Romi teaches people how to figure out what they really want, what their time is worth and exactly where to spend it, what to delegate and delete, how to tame technology, how to cut toxic people out of their life and more ways to live the full, focused and less-overwhelming life we all deserve.

## 🦴 Take Action 🦴

Like with exercise, when it comes to reducing stress, you've got lots of options. Some of them are relatively easy, like getting out into nature more. Others, like dealing more effectively with problems and cutting an addiction to multitasking, may require more time and effort. Making stress reduction a non-negotiable priority is the first step.

Focus on creating these healthy habits in your life by working on them every day. Once they become part of your life, they'll be easier to do. When that happens, build on that success and pick another one.

**Write down three things now that you'll commit to doing to de-stress:**

1._____

2._____

3._____

## Chapter 10

# Catch Some ZZZs

N o one enjoys dragging through the day because of exhaustion. Unfortunately, as people get older sleeping difficulties are more common, and our society in general has become more sleep deprived than ever. When we don't get enough it wreaks havoc on our health and destroys our bones. Adequate sleep is required to learn new tasks, to keep your immune system strong, to deal with stress and to have enough energy to do everything we want to do.[1]

Simply put: sleep is essential. And when we're getting enough, we have more energy to exercise and are more likely to eat healthy, which are both important for protecting our bones. The optimal amount of sleep for adults is 7-8 hours a night.[2] Yet 20% of adults sleep less than 6.5 hours a night.[3,4] Over the last century, the number of hours people sleep has decreased by 25% and as many as 70 million Americans now suffer with chronic sleep problems![5]

If you're sleeping less than an average of six hours a night, you're two times more likely to suffer high blood pressure, four times more likely to suffer major depression and 30% more likely to die compared to those who get enough sleep.[6] Stud-

Studies show that not getting enough sleep reduces quality of life as much as having congestive heart failure and major depressive disorders.[6,7]

As for your bones, sleep deprivation is associated with significantly lower bone mineral density and increased osteoporosis risk.[8] And since not getting enough sleep decreases your balance, coordination and reaction time, it also increases your risk for falls and fractures.

Sleep issues are fixable, so let's talk about what might be preventing you from getting enough ZZZs and how to fix the problem.

As for your bones, sleep deprivation is associated with significantly lower bone mineral density and increased osteoporosis risk.

## Sleep Meds

People frequently try over the counter (OTC) or prescription sleep medications. OTC antihistamines that contain the drug diphenhydramine, which is the active ingredient in Benadryl, are popular. While they may work as a short-term fix, the body can build up a tolerance to the medications. The longer you take them, the less likely they are to be effective.

The most common drugs for sleep are the "Z-drugs." These are in the category called benzodiazepine or benzodiazepine-like medications. They go by names such as Halcion, Prosom, Ambien, Lunesta and Sonata.

The Z-drugs are typically used for insomnia. However, while they can increase sleep *quantity*, they don't increase sleep *quality* and they have serious side effects. They can decrease daytime alertness and cause dizziness and lightheadedness. They can also increases the risk for accidents, falls, cognitive impairment and cancer.[9,10] People over 60 have a harder time breaking down and eliminating Z-drugs. This means they can end up with high amounts of the medication in their bodies that increases their risks for dangerous side effects. One study concluded that these drugs may be associated with half a million deaths per year.[11]

A newer class of drugs is called orexin receptor antagonists. In 2015 the FDA approved the first medication in this class, named Suvorexant (Belsomra). Belsomra decreases the amount of time it takes to fall asleep by about 10 minutes and can increase sleep duration by up to 20 minutes.[12] But the side effects are scary. Both Belsomra and Z-drugs have been shown to cause amnesia, anxiety, hallucinations, "sleep-driving" (driving while not fully awake) and other activities while asleep—preparing and eating food, making phone calls or having sex—without remembering the events. They can also cause impairment the next day after taking them and increase thoughts of suicide.

> Belsomra and Z-drugs have been shown to cause amnesia, anxiety, hallucinations, "sleep-driving" (driving while not fully awake) and other activities while asleep—preparing and eating food, making phone calls, or having sex—without remembering the events.

## What Else You Can Do

In my opinion, it's much safer to explore fixing your sleep without medications using nutrients that nourish your body, promote healthy sleep and by getting rid of "sleep destroyers."

### Technology

One major reason people aren't sleeping enough is technology, including the centuries-old lightbulb and our now always-connected, 24/7 addiction to screens. It used to be that when it was dark, it was bedtime. There wasn't a way to simply flip a switch and have as much light as we wanted. And our addiction to our computers, smartphones and tablets are a compelling and dangerous distraction from sleep.

Smartphones are small computers, and the technology that we carry around in our pockets or purses is incredibly powerful—more powerful than the first supercomputer. The ability for us to instantly access research on any topic on a whim, to work seamlessly with people in different cities, states or countries, to check movie times and buy movie tickets or make restaurant reservations with a few taps of our fingers is incredible. It's changed our expectations and how we work, play and unwind.

But there's a downside. If you've made health a priority, which I hope you have, total health means more than exercising and eating healthy. Total health also means understanding the impact technology has on your health and your children.

We now know that our devices affect our brain chemistry and alter hormone levels. They can increase the amount of dopamine secreted and deplete melatonin. These changes have serious effects on our mood and sleep cycles and can literally make you sick.

Gaming, television and social media companies understand this and create entire products based on dopamine. In his book, *Hooked: How to Build Habit-Forming Products*, Nir Eyal discusses how companies engineer user experiences to profit from our brain's natural love affair with dopamine. When you're working on a smartphone or a tablet, and you're tapping away, scrolling and swiping, you're getting hits of dopamine, a feel-good hormone.

This experience isn't much different from snorting cocaine. Cocaine is so addictive because it floods the brain with dopamine. Once it wears off, the dopamine levels are lower than they were before, and people reach for the drug again to get their dopamine fix.

Anyone with a smartphone knows how addictive they are. How many times have you compulsively grabbed yours because you felt anxious after not swiping or scrolling for a bit? I have. That could be the dopamine talking.

If you work on your tablet or your smartphone in bed at night, we also know that it decreases your brain's ability to secrete melatonin. Melatonin is a hormone that helps regulate sleep and is the trigger that starts putting us to sleep. It also helps modulate circadian rhythms, the energy and rhythm of day and night.

A 2015 clinical trial published in the *Proceedings of the*

*National Academy of Sciences* showed just how damaging these devices can be to our health. The researchers studied the effects of reading an eBook before bed and discovered that it decreased melatonin more than 55%.[13]

The effects on how volunteers slept and their physical functioning the next day were alarming. It took volunteers an additional 10 minutes to fall asleep compared with people who were reading a hard-copy book before bed. That doesn't seem like a lot to me. And when I read it, I thought, "What's the big deal?" But then I looked at what happened the next day. For folks who were on their devices before bed, it took them *hours longer* to feel fully awake in the morning and attain the same level of alertness compared to people reading the old-fashioned way.

Working on your tablet or your smartphone in bed at night can create difficulty falling asleep and keep you from getting the high-quality sleep your body needs. Then you wake up tired. And when you're tired, what do you do? You start craving starchy, sugary foods, which puts you on a roller coaster of a blood-sugar high, followed by a crash and craving more sugar. It also creates dopamine and cortisol regulation issues. That's why you find yourself reaching for your smartphone again to get a hit of feel-good dopamine because sleep deprivation decreases your mood.

So put your phone away at night and make your bedroom a device-free zone. It can help you sleep better, leading to a host of health benefits. And it can also help you connect with your partner. Make your bedroom about sleep and connecting and make it free of technology. Instead of scrolling, read a book or magazine. Or better yet, connect with your partner and improve your relationship. I talk more about the importance of social support in Chapter 12.

## Social Jetlag

I can't overstate the importance of sleep consistency. Fitbit creates wearable activity monitors. Because of how popular the devices are, the company has access to an amazing amount of data. Fitbit did a study of six billion data points generated by its customers. It was the largest data analysis in the history of sleep science.[14,15] The biggest finding was the link between sleep quality and sleep consistency. They discovered that going to bed at the same time every night is the biggest predictor of healthy sleep.

People often go to bed at roughly the same time during the week. But when the weekend comes, they tend to stay up later. This bedtime inconsistency can lead to difficulty sleeping. If somebody goes out on a Friday night, and then again on Saturday, and they're up until 12:00 or 1:00 or 2:00 in the morning, they're inducing what Fitbit calls Social Jetlag.

Then when they try to go to sleep earlier on Sunday and Monday, their body was trained over the weekend that it's too early for bed. It's as if they took an airplane to a different time zone and have real jet

Sleep consistency— going to bed every night and training the body when it's time to go to sleep—is crucial for high-quality sleep.

lag, but this jet lag was caused by their social life.

Sleep consistency—going to bed every night and training the body when it's time to go to sleep—is crucial for high-quality sleep.

### Your Mid-Afternoon Coffee Pick-Me-Up

More than 80% of Americans drink coffee. And while it may be America's favorite pick-me-up, it's possible to have too much of a good thing. Drinking coffee in the afternoon or evening can keep you tossing and turning at night. If you find yourself having a hard time falling asleep and you're drinking coffee late in the day, stop it.

Mid-afternoon energy slumps are typically due to low blood sugar. Instead of reaching for caffeine, reach for a snack with protein, which is one of the best ways to regulate blood sugar and get a boost of energy the healthy way. For a list of healthy protein snacks, see the table in the Appendix.

### Acid Reflux

Acid reflux, also called gastroesophageal reflux disorder (GERD), is better known as plain old heartburn. Most people think of heartburn as a burning in their chest or back of their throat. While heartburn creates those problems, you can also have heartburn without burning. Heartburn can show up as a dry, hacking cough. Whether it's a burning sensation or a dry hacking cough, the symptoms of heartburn are worse when laying down and improve when standing up. Heartburn can make it hard to fall asleep, make it difficult to get into a deep sleep and wake you up during the night.

The conventional approach to helping people with heartburn is to recommend antacids like Tums or acid-blocker medications like Prilosec, Zantac, Nexium or Prevacid. Antacids work by buffering the acid using calcium carbonate. Acid-blockers work by decreasing the stomach's production of acid.

Neither one cures the problem, and both have potential side effects. Antacids can cause constipation and as I discussed in detail in Chapter 5, acid-blockers damage bone and increase your risk for osteoporosis and fractures. Acid blockers are also associated with increased risks for stomach cancer and dementia.[16-18]

Natural approaches can provide benefits without the dangerous side effects. An excellent place to start is to investigate whether the underlying cause is dietary. Some foods are known heartburn triggers. If you're experiencing heartburn, try cutting the following foods out of your diet for a few days and see if your health and sleep improve:

- alcohol, particularly red wine
- black pepper, garlic, raw onions, and other spicy foods
- chocolate
- citrus fruits and products, such as lemons, oranges and orange juice
- coffee and caffeinated drinks, including tea and soda
- peppermint
- tomatoes

## Snoring

When air can't flow smoothly through your nose to the back of your mouth and down your trachea to your lungs, it can cause snoring. Not only can it create problems with your partner by waking them up (just ask my wife), it can also wake you up or keep you from reaching the deep, restorative stage of sleep your body needs. This can leave you feeling tired and dragging through your day.

And while there are lots of companies selling anti-snoring promises—strips that attach to your nose, mouthpieces that thrust your jaw forward, devices that stick into your nose and adjustable beds—changing your diet is an easy, no-cost approach that too often gets overlooked.

I'm speaking from first-hand experience. For years I struggled with snoring. I tried every device I could find. Some would work for a while, but then stop. Others would help but the device was so uncomfortable that I couldn't sleep. And still others didn't work at all.

Then I realized dairy was creating inflammation, post-nasal drip and congestion. When I'd eat cheese or ice cream, my snoring would get worse. When I avoided those foods, I wasn't congested and, lo-and-behold, my snoring wasn't as bad. If you have post-nasal drip or congestion, try eliminating dairy for a few days and see if this helps.

I was surprised to discover one of my most problematic things wasn't a food at all; it was coffee. I realized that when I drank coffee, I got a bit phlegmy. So I quit. Three days later I realized I had zero post-nasal drip. Not only was I breathing easier, but my snoring decreased by 75% according to my wife and we were able to sleep in the same bed again without me waking her up all night sawing wood.

Even when one thing helps your snoring, it still may come back. As I mentioned, I've experimented with lots of devices. Three that I've found most helpful are snore strips, nose vent plugs and Smart Nora®. Nose vent plugs are nasal dilators that have vents cut into them for airflow. Smart Nora contains a device you slip beneath your pillow. When you snore, it detects the sounds and inflates, which adjusts your neck and head automatically into a new position to open your airway and stop the snoring.

Your snoring might be caused by sleep apnea. If your partner says you seem to stop breathing or gasp for air during the night, or if dietary changes or devices don't work, consult a sleep specialist to help you understand if a sleep apnea machine might help.

**Alcohol**

Alcohol can damage sleep in many ways. It can make acid reflux worse. While it's a sedative and can decrease the time it takes people to fall asleep, for many people it creates a rebound effect, waking them up in the middle of the night.

You may be waking up in the middle of the night from alcohol for a different reason. Alcohol is a diuretic and increases the kidney's urine production. And many people who get woken up in the middle of the night have a hard time falling back to sleep.

Alcohol also can increase your snoring, which can decrease sleep quality and leave you feeling tired and groggy in the morning.

### Poor Blood Sugar Control

While low blood sugar can create a mid-afternoon drop in energy, it can also wake you up from a deep sleep. When your blood sugar drops, hormones are released to breakdown stored sugars. The hormones, cortisol and epinephrine, not only free up sugar for your body to use, they also wake you up.

One way to help control your blood sugar for a better night's sleep is to avoid eating sugary desserts and snacks. You can also try eating about ten grams of protein before bed, since protein is one of the best ways to help regulate blood sugar. For a list of healthy protein snacks, see the protein table in the Appendix.

### Waking Up to Pee

If you're waking up at night to go to the bathroom, one simple solution is to make sure you stop drinking liquids earlier in the evening. Stop all liquids at least three hours before bed unless you need a little water to take medications or dietary supplements. If that doesn't do the trick, try four hours before bed.

### Stress, the Sleep Killer

People who have difficulty falling asleep or staying asleep may be struggling with increased stress. Increased stress can cause insomnia and poor sleep, including a whole host of other health issues. In Chapter 9 you made a list of things you'll do to destress. But when it comes specifically to improving sleep, here are some effective strategies that can help.

- **Get it out of your head.** If your mind is racing at night with everything you have to do the next day, write it all down before bed. This can help you drift off to sleep knowing that you have a handle on all of it.
- **Meditate.** Meditation has phenomenal health benefits. One of them is to reduce stress, which can help you sleep better. Even if you have zero experience, there are some excellent meditation apps for your smartphone that can help you. While you can meditate longer, just ten minutes once daily can have wonderful benefits.
- **Exercise.** Exercise decreases cortisol and can improve your sleep. In one study, aerobic exercise—walking, stationary bike or using a treadmill—four days a week for thirty minutes each time improved sleep in women 55 years old and up who had insomnia.[19]
- **Get into nature.** Taking a walk outside or going for a hike reduces stress and improves mood.

These simple, natural solutions can have profound, positive impacts on your sleep and improve your energy and quality of life.

## Medications that Cause Insomnia

Evaluating your medications is important, because many can affect sleep and create insomnia and other sleep disorders.[20-22] If you're taking medications and experiencing difficulty sleeping, increased daytime fatigue or decreased mood, check with your pharmacist or healthcare provider to see if the prescriptions might be creating the problem.

Some of the most commonly prescribed drugs with these side effects are:

- **Beta blockers.** Used to treat high blood pressure (hypertension), arrhythmia, heart failure, chest pain (angina), heart attacks, migraine headaches and certain tremors, they include Acebutolol (Sectral), Atenolol (Tenormin), Bisoprolol (Zebeta), Metoprolol (Lopressor, Toprol-XL), Nadolol (Corgard), Nebivolol (Bystolic), Propranolol (Inderal LA, InnoPran XL). These drugs cause insomnia because they deplete melatonin.
- **Alpha agonist.** These are also high blood pressure medications and include Catapres (Clonidine), Doxazosin, Phentolamine, Phenoxybenzamine, Prazosin, Terazosin, Tolazoline
- **Mixed alpha + beta blockers** go by the names Bucindolol, Carbedilol, Labetalol
- **Anti-inflammatory and immune modulating steroids.** These are prescribed to treat autoimmune diseases such as Lupus and Rheumatoid Arthritis. They're sold under the names of prednisone, prednisolone and methylpred-

nisone. In addition to causing insomnia, these drugs cause osteoporosis and fractures.

- **Antidepressant medications.** Many antidepressants cause insomnia; in fact, there are too many to list. If you're taking an antidepressant medication and are having difficulty sleeping, speak to your healthcare provider or pharmacist to see if sleep disruption is a known side effect.

## Poor Sleep Hygiene

Sleep hygiene is about ensuring your sleep environment promotes sleep and doesn't keep you awake. To help you get better sleep, make sure your bedroom is:

- **Dark.** Light can keep the body in a lighter sleep state and can signal the body that it's time to wake up. Some people like wearing sleep masks to keep the light out if they are particularly sensitive.
- **At the optimal temperature for sleep.** While this can vary from person to person, the optimal temperature for most people seems to be 69- or 70-degrees Fahrenheit.
- **Quiet or has white noise.** Some people find they sleep better with some background noise. You can download an app on your smartphone that will play white noise, such as the sound of wind, rain or waves.

## Pain and Discomfort

Pain and discomfort make it hard to find a comfortable position to sleep. The body naturally tries to find a position that minimizes the pain. That may mean laying on your back, stomach or side. It may mean sleeping with a pillow between your legs or stretching your arm up under your pillow.

Understanding the cause of the pain and discomfort is important in finding the best solution. The conventional, pharmacological approach to pain is to recommend people take pain medications, such as Celebrex, Tylenol (Acetaminophen) or Ibuprofen. While these drugs can provide excellent relief, they are not without serious side effects when taken long-term. Acetaminophen is the number one cause of non-infectious liver failure, which is liver failure not caused by an infection such as hepatitis.

Musculoskeletal pain is a major cause of sleep issues for many people. The list of potential integrative and natural options available for pain is too long to include here. I recommend you consider working with a naturopathic doctor, a chiropractic doctor or integrative medical doctor to address any underlying issues.

One reason many people have trouble falling and staying asleep is because of tight muscles. Stretching such as gentle yoga, an Epsom salt soak in a hot bath or relaxing in a hot tub can all help relieve muscle tension.

The dietary supplements magnesium and gamma amino butyric acid (GABA) can also help relax the body for sleep. GABA relaxes the nervous system while magnesium is a gentle muscle relaxer.

## ♫ Take Action ♫

To improve sleep, I've found that a combination of approaches gives the best results. Each person is different, so be patient as you try different things and discover what works for you. Know that over time what you need may also change.

Some strategies are relatively easy, like simply drinking less at night before you go to bed, turning the thermostat down to a comfortable sleeping temperature and eliminating foods that can cause snoring. Others will take more time and patience. As with all areas of your health, I encourage you to see this as a process that you will keep exploring until you discover what works best for you.

**Now, write down three things that you'll commit to right away to improve your sleep:**

1. _____

2. _____

3. _____

Once you've accomplished the things on your list, write down three more and get to work on those. Keep doing this until you've figured out the best combination that gives you the sleep you need.

1. _____

2. _____

3. _____

## Chapter 11

# Dietary Supplements

Dietary supplements for bone health are big business. According to the dietary supplement industry publication, *Nutraceuticals World*, the bone and joint dietary supplement market was $250 million in the U.S. alone in 2015. As the population ages and more people are affected by osteoporosis, the market continues to grow.

But for all the hard-earned money people are spending to protect their bones, are they getting their money's worth? Are you protected as much as possible, or as much as you think you are?

Understanding how to evaluate research on nutrients and dietary supplements is important for helping you make the best possible decisions for your health. So, let's review what the science says for the most common bone-building nutrients.

## Calcium and Vitamin D

When people think about a bone health dietary supplement, the two nutrients that most often come to mind are calcium and vitamin D. The FDA allows supplement companies to claim that "Adequate calcium and vitamin D throughout life, as part of a well-balanced diet, may reduce the risk of osteoporosis." And doctors routinely recommend these two nutrients. But do they reduce fracture risk? When combined, calcium and vitamin D decrease fracture risk by 10-23%.[1,2]

**Calcium and vitamin D decrease fracture risk by 10-23%.**

Calcium carbonate is the most common form of calcium in supplements, but this mineral is poorly absorbed and can cause constipation.[3] Absorbing calcium carbonate requires stomach acid to separate the calcium from the carbonate. As we age, however, low stomach acid becomes more common. An estimated 10–21% of people 60-69 years old, 31% of those 70-79 years old, and 37% of those 80 years and older have low or no stomach acid.[4] Stomach acid production is also low if you take acid blocking medications, have an untreated *H. pylori* infection, have an autoimmune condition or you're chronically stressed.

On the other hand, calcium citrate, calcium malate and calcium as an amino acid chelate are absorbed much easier than calcium carbonate. For example, the absorption of calcium citrate is approximately 24% higher than calcium carbonate. And when stomach acid is low, you absorb 200% more calcium from calcium citrate compared to calcium carbonate.[5] Finally, if you struggle with calcium oxalate, cystine or uric acid kidney stones, calcium citrate is the preferred form since citrate prevents the formation of these types of kidney stones.[6]

The US Recommended Daily Amount (RDA) of calcium for women is 1,000 mg per day until they reach 50 years old, then increases to 1,200 mg. For men up to 70 years old, it's 1,000 mg per day, then 1,200 mg after that. It's important to understand that the US RDA is a general target thought to provide adequate nutrition for most people. Your calcium amount doesn't have to match it exactly. In fact, your health-care provider may recommend a different amount based on her assessment of your needs.

While you can get more calcium than the US RDA, you don't want to take too much. Clinical guidelines from the Bone Health and Osteoporosis Foundation and the American Society for Preventive Cardiology recommend people consume less than 2,000-2,5000 mg of total calcium per day. This is from all sources—diet and dietary supplements—and matches the recommendation from the National Academy of Medicine.[7]

For most people, how much calcium they should get from supplements depends on their diet. On average, American women get about 800 mg of calcium per day from diet and men get about 1,000 mg per day.[8] For many women, therefore, taking an extra 400 mg of calcium as a dietary supplement is enough to reach the US RDA for calcium. However, even if women take 1,000 mg of calcium as a dietary supplement, most will still be below the upper limit of 2,000-2,500 mg set by the National Academy of Medicine. For others, like folks who don't eat dairy, they may need more.

But you don't have to eat dairy to get enough calcium. Plants are a great source. When you follow my Osteoporosis Diet in Chapter 7, you'll naturally be eating more plants and getting more calcium. If you want to know how much calcium you're consuming and which foods are excellent sources for this important mineral, the Calcium Content of Foods table in Appendix B is a handy reference. It's also available to download at nbiheatlh.com/osteobook.

Additionally, healthy bones depend on having enough vitamin D. This powerful nutrient regulates more than 200 genes and is one of the most important molecules for your health. Since vitamin D affects so many genes, it's not surprising that this nutrient helps protect you from a whole host of problems. Vitamin D can help you fight infections; help protect against diabetes, heart disease, cancer, asthma, depression, autoimmune diseases like multiple sclerosis (MS) and rheumatoid arthritis (RA); and boost your immune system. Vitamin D helps regulate calcium and phosphorous balance, promotes healthy inflammation balance and supports bone, immune, colon and breast health.

Vitamin D is so important that your body produces it from sunlight. When the ultraviolet B (UVB) rays in sunlight hit your body, it converts cholesterol in your skin to pre-vitamin D.[9] The liver then converts pre-vitamin D to vitamin D2, which then undergoes its final transformation to vitamin D3 in the kidneys.[10]

Despite the fact that your body produces its own vitamin D3, deficiency is rampant.[11,12] According to two studies that evaluated vitamin D levels, about 40% of adults and 70% of

**Despite the fact that your body produces its own vitamin D3, deficiency is rampant.**

children are deficient in this crucial nutrient.[13,14] People with malabsorption issues, such as Crohn's disease, Ulcerative Colitis and Celiac disease, and the elderly have even higher risks for vitamin D deficiency.

Several things explain why so many people lack vitamin D. These days we just don't get enough steady sunlight, and when we do, we're either covered up or we slather ourselves with sunblock, preventing UVB from penetrating our skin. To prevent Vitamin D deficiency, it takes 15-20 minutes of sunshine daily with more than 40% of your skin exposed.[9]

If you live in the northern hemisphere above 37 degrees north latitude, the sun in the winter never gets high enough to stimulate our own vitamin D production.[15] Where exactly is that? Thirty-seven degrees north latitude is an imaginary line that passes through California (near Santa Cruz), Nevada, southern Utah, northern Arizona, along the Colorado/New Mexico border, and through the Kansas/Oklahoma border, Missouri, southern Illinois, Kentucky and Virginia. So, if you live in those areas, or north of them, in the winter your risk for vitamin D deficiency is higher than your neighbors to the south.

Darker skin, which contains relatively more melanin than lighter skin, slows the production of vitamin D. Similarly, aging reduces skin vitamin D production. Common glass in home or car windows and clothing all reduce UVB radiation exposure, even in summer months.

Vitamin D should be on everyone's radar. Not having enough vitamin D has been associated with increased risks of deadly cancers, cardiovascular disease, multiple sclerosis, depression, schizophrenia, rheumatoid arthritis and insulin-dependent diabetes.[16,17] Vitamin D is so important to health that a 2008 study found low blood levels were associated with double the risk of dying from any cause.[18] This trend was confirmed by a larger study that showed supplementing with vitamin D3 reduced cancer deaths.[19]

For bone health, making sure you have enough vitamin D is crucial. Higher vitamin D levels are associated with increased bone mineral density and reduced fracture risk, especially as you get older.[20] To reduce the risks for falls and fractures, a person's Vitamin D blood concentration should be 30-44 nanograms per milliliter (ng/mL). Above 30 ng/mL, nonvertebral fractures decrease by 20% and hip fractures by 18%. Similarly, the greatest decrease in the risk for falling is seen when someone's vitamin D level is about 30 ng/mL and dying from any cause was reduced when the blood level was 40-48 ng/mL.[21] But even higher might be better. For additional health benefits such as immune support, clinical trials and meta-analyses concluded that an optimal range appears to be about 50-60 ng/mL.[21,22]

Most healthy adults can increase their vitamin D blood level to 30-44 ng/mL when taking a daily supplement containing 1,800 to 4,000 IU (45-100 mcg) of vitamin D3.[21] But to get your levels higher, you'll likely need to take more. Multiple studies concluded that vitamin D levels increase by about 1 ng/

> For bone health, making sure you have enough vitamin D is crucial.

mL for every 100 IU (2.5 mcg) of vitamin D3.[23,24] Therefore, to get vitamin D into the optimal range of 50-60 ng/mL, you may need to take at least 5,000 IU (125 mcg) of Vitamin D3 per day.

> **To get vitamin D into the optimal range of 50-60 ng/mL, you may need to take at least 5,000 IU (125 mcg) of Vitamin D3 per day.**

It takes about five to six months to reach a steady state, at which point your vitamin D level remains fairly constant.[25] Many clinicians recommend testing your vitamin D every few months to make sure it's approaching an optimal level and to know whether you need to adjust the dose.

More than 20 publications conclude that there is no association between harm and intakes of 10,000 IU (250 mcg) per day.[21,26-28] In fact, an expert committee of the Food and Nutrition Board at the US National Academies of Sciences, Engineering and Medicine (NASEM) concluded that toxicity is unlikely at intakes below 10,000 IU daily.[29]

While it's important to work with your healthcare provider to determine the optimal dose and blood levels for you, Vitamin D toxicity doesn't generally occur until serum vitamin D reaches 100-150 ng/mL.[30,31]

## Vitamin K2 (MK4 and MK7)

MK4 and MK7 are two types of natural vitamin K2 commercially available in dietary supplements to promote bone health. MK4 is the major form of vitamin K that accumulates throughout the body—in the testes, pancreas, kidneys, brain and arteries.[32,33] In fact, tissues that accumulate high amounts of MK4 have a remarkable capacity to convert up to 90% of the available K1 into MK4.[34,35] This hints at MK4s wide-ranging benefits beyond bone health.

There are two crucial questions to ask when considering a bone health dietary supplement that contains MK4 or MK7. They are:

1. Has the form of vitamin K2 (MK4 or MK7) been shown in studies to reduce fractures?
2. Has the dose of the vitamin in the product been shown in studies to reduce fractures?

For these two questions, the research overwhelmingly supports the MK4 form of vitamin K2 in the amount of 45 mg/day. MK7 has never been shown in studies to reduce fractures. The U.S. National Library of Medicine's PubMed database, the definitive clinical research database in the country, only lists five clinical trials that studied the effect of MK7 on bone health in people with osteoporosis, and none of those studies evaluated MK7's ability to reduce fractures as a study outcome.

In contrast, the benefits of MK4 for bone health in people with osteoporosis have been studied in 28 human clinical trials with more than 7,000 people. Not only have researchers repeatedly concluded that MK4 supports healthy bone laboratory markers and bone density, but seven clinical trials specifically evaluated MK4's ability to maintain strong bones by looking at fractures.

In fact, MK4 (45 mg/day) has been so well researched that since 1995 it's been approved by the Ministry of Health in Japan for the treatment of osteoporosis and bone pain caused by osteoporosis.[36] In the U.S., however, the FDA has not approved MK4 to diagnose, treat, prevent or cure any disease.

Clinical trials using 45 mg per day of MK4 show this dose, and only this amount, promotes healthy bone density and maintains strong bones as indicated by—in one study—up to 87% fewer fractures independent of the number of falls.[37] Since different clinical trials can come up with different results, pooling data from many clinical trials into what researchers call a *meta-analysis* can provide a clearer picture. Fortunately for us, two groups of researchers did exactly that for MK4.

A review of clinical trials published in 2006 concluded that MK4 decreases vertebral fractures by 60% and all non-vertebral fractures by 76%.[38] A more recent study came to similar conclusions. A 2015 meta-analysis concluded that taking MK4 (45 mg/day) reduced overall fractures by 53% in postmenopausal women with osteoporosis.[39]

> A review of clinical trials published in 2006 concluded that MK4 decreases vertebral fractures by 60% and all nonvertebral fractures by 76%.

In clinical trials, MK4 (45 mg daily) has proven helpful in promoting bone health and maintaining strong bones in people struggling with bone loss from:

• menopause (postmenopausal osteoporosis)[36-38,40-42]

- corticosteroids (e.g., prednisone, dexamethasone, prednisolone)[43-46]
- anorexia nervosa[47]
- cirrhosis of the liver[48]
- decreased mobility from stroke[49]
- primary biliary cirrhosis[50]
- androgen deprivation therapy (ADT) using leuprolide[51]

In addition to maintaining bone strength, only MK4 has also been shown to promote healthy bone marrow and support brain, liver and immune health. Bone marrow creates red blood cells, white blood cells and platelets. Red blood cells carry oxygen throughout your body. White blood cells power your immune system. And platelets are required for healthy blood clotting. All these cells are produced by stem cells in your bone marrow, and MK4 supports healthy stem cell production.[52]

> MK4 has also been shown to promote healthy bone marrow and support brain, liver and immune health.

In the brain, MK4 accumulates in specific regions, such as the:

- midbrain (involved in eye movement, vision and processing sounds)
- pons (generates respiratory rhythm and breathing)
- cerebellum (helps maintain balance)
- olfactory bulb (processes your sense of smell)
- thalamus (regulates consciousness and alertness)

• hippocampus (plays a major role in memory and learning)
• striatum (important for movement)

Since MK4 accumulates in these areas, it suggests this nutrient is the active form of vitamin K in the brain and may have powerful benefit for brain health and nerve function.[53,54] Finally, MK4 supports liver health by maintaining healthy cells. MK4 inhibits NF-kB and matrix metalloproteinase (MMP) in liver cells.[55,56] NF-kB increases inflammation, so lowering NF-kB helps promote healthy inflammation balance. MMP plays a key role in regulating the immune system and lowering MMP activity is associated with improved immune health and healthy cell structure.[57]

MK4 is not only effective, it's safe at 45 mg/day and even at higher amounts. Published research has documented the safety in humans of 135 mg/day of MK4, and 250 mg/kg body weight per day in rats.[40,58] These studies also concluded that MK4 does not increase the risk for blood clots. To put the animal dose in perspective, if a typical adult weighs 150 pounds and takes 250 mg of MK4 per kg body weight, they'd consume 17,000 mg (17 kilograms!) of MK4. That amount is nearly 380 times more than the 45 mg/day used in the clinical trials for bone health.

Published studies have followed more than 7,000 volunteers for up to six years without any dangerous side effects from taking 45 mg and higher of MK4 daily. The only known exception to MK4's safety is when people are taking the medication Warfarin (Coumadin). This blood thinner works by blocking the ability of vitamin K to promote blood clotting. When someone on warfarin takes vitamin K it counteracts the medication. For other types of blood thinners, like Lovenox (enoxaparin), that do not work by interfering with vitamin K, MK4 do not interact negatively with the drug. Similarly, MK4 is safe to take with all osteoporosis medications.

The overwhelming research supports the safety of MK4 and that it's the only form of vitamin K shown in basic research and clinical trials to demonstrate all these benefits.

## Collagen

Collagen is the most abundant protein in the body. It's the scaffolding that holds your body together. In fact, the origin of the word collagen is the Greek word Kolla, or glue. It's so strong that even the smallest building blocks of collagen are five to ten times stronger than steel.[59] Collagen provides structure to skin, bones, tendons, cartilage, connective tissue, arteries, muscles and teeth; and helps keep them healthy and strong.

Although your body has at least 16 types of collagen, Type I collagen is the most common. Ninety percent of your body's collagen is Type I collagen. Type I collagen also makes up 90% of the non-mineral part of bones.[60] Another common one is Type III collagen.

For dietary supplements, collagen is broken down in a process called hydrolysis. That's why you'll often see "hydrolyzed collagen" on product labels. Research indicates that hydrolyzed collagen is safe, highly absorbable and supports healthy bone metabolism and bone strength.[61,62]

While there are no studies that looked at fracture risk with collagen, a review of over 60 scientific studies on collagen found that supplementing with collagen peptides promotes healthy tissue regeneration, collagen synthesis and supports healthy joints, bone density and skin.[63] Animal studies have also given excellent results. In one study, rats with fractured femurs (the thigh bone) healed faster when they were fed hydrolyzed collagen.[64]

When collagen degrades, bone breaks down and collagen fragments are released. One of these is C-terminal telopeptide (CTX). It can be measured in the urine and serum (the liquid part of blood). One benefit of measuring CTX is that it shows changes much faster than can be detected on a bone density test.

High levels of CTX have been shown to predict fracture risk in postmenopausal women.[65] A 2000 study followed 435 women ages 31-89 years old for an average of five years. The highest urinary and serum CTX results were associated with increased fracture risk. If someone also had low bone mineral density and low levels of estrogen, their risk was even higher.[66] A different study published the same year found that elevated CTX is strongly associated with fractures in elderly women.[67]

The International Osteoporosis Foundation (IOF) and International Federation of Clinical Chemistry (IFCC) recommend the CTX blood test as a marker to predict fracture risk and to monitor osteoporosis treatment.[65]

The great news is that a clinical trial showed that taking collagen can lower CTX. This indicates that collagen reduces bone breakdown. In a study of 51 postmenopausal women with osteopenia, CTX was decreased by taking five grams of collagen peptides daily, plus calcium and vitamin D3, for three months. CTX decreased almost four times more in people taking collagen, plus calcium and vitamin D3, compared to people only taking calcium and vitamin D3. In those women taking collagen, CTX decreased 11.4% compared to 3.5% in the control group. This implies that significantly less bone was breaking down when taking collagen.[68]

**Collagen reduces bone breakdown.**

## Boron

Boron is a trace mineral that was first discovered in 1910 as being required for plant development and health. In 1985 researchers discovered that humans also require boron in tiny amounts. However, there are no studies showing that boron improves bone mineral density, decreases bone loss or decreases fractures. Multivitamin and mineral supplements will often contain this nutrient anyway. But for building stronger bones and reducing fractures, there are no clinical trials supporting its use in a bone support dietary supplement.

## Melatonin

Melatonin is a popular dietary supplement for sleep. Your body naturally produces melatonin in the pineal gland in your brain and in your gut. While most people only think about melatonin for helping them to sleep, melatonin also helps your bones. Melatonin suppresses bone loss and promotes new bone formation.[69]

The hypothesis that melatonin might be helpful in people with osteoporosis was tested in a 2015 study with 81 postmenopausal women with osteopenia.[70] This placebo-controlled, randomized clinical trial had women taking one mg of melatonin, three mg of melatonin or a placebo at bedtime for one year. After one year they found that BMD significantly increased in women taking both one mg and three mg of melatonin, with the higher dose providing greater benefit. In women taking three mg of melatonin, femoral neck BMD increased 2.3% and the spine BMD increased 3.6%. However, BMD did not increase at any other sites (eg, the forearms or wrists). Additionally, the researchers did not evaluate whether taking melatonin also reduced fracture risk. Hopefully, future research will test melatonin in people with osteoporosis and, most importantly, evaluate whether melatonin reduces fractures.

## Strontium

Several rigorous clinical trials have evaluated strontium for its bone building effects. Strontium ranelate (SR) is a form of strontium salt from ranelic acid patented by a French company. SR is the only form of strontium that has ever been studied in clinical trials and is not available in the US. Instead, dietary supplements in the US contain strontium citrate, which has never been shown in any clinical trials to support healthy bone density or reduce fractures.

SR is an approved osteoporosis treatment in most of Europe, but not in the US. Studies in rats concluded that SR incorporates into bone, decreases bone loss and can increase bone density.[71] A laboratory study determined that SR can also promote osteoblast production.[72] Clinical trials have shown that taking 500-2000 mg per day of SR can decrease vertebral fractures by 23% to 49%, as well as increase bone mineral density.[73,74]

Despite these studies, you may want to think twice before taking strontium for several reasons. First, while strontium citrate has been shown to incorporate into bones,[75] strontium creates false bone density test results. Since strontium is heavier than calcium, x-rays from a bone density scan bounce off the strontium to a greater degree than calcium and change what's called the "refractive index." Unless the radiologist understands this and uses a mathematical calculation to correct for this, the bone density scan will be inaccurate.[73] Since radiologists are not taught this in medical school or residency, even if you tell them that you're taking strontium, the radiologist most likely won't know how to correct for it to provide an accurate result.

Strontium has also been linked to an increased risk for dangerous blood clots, called venous thromboembolism (VTE), blood clots in the lungs (pulmonary thromboembolism) and heart attacks. According to a 2014 comparison of European regulatory data and publications for strontium (in the form of strontium ranelate), "the number of fractures prevented by strontium use is similar to the number of extra cases of venous thromboembolism, pulmonary embolism and myocardial infarction caused by strontium."[76] While studies showed strontium reduces fracture risk, it's just as effective at increasing your risk for a potentially deadly blood clot and heart attack.

## Magnesium

Magnesium may play a role in promoting bone health. Yet only one small clinical trial, conducted in 1993, has been published on the ability of magnesium to build bone.[77] This study concluded that taking a few hundred milligrams daily of magnesium (as magnesium hydroxide, one of the least absorbable forms of magnesium) may increase bone density. However, a more recent study evaluating data from 73,684 postmenopausal women concluded that magnesium intake had no effect on fracture risk.[78]

I've seen on the internet claims that calcium and magnesium are required for calcium absorption and magnesium must therefore be in a bone health supplement. In nearly two decades of research and clinical work, I have yet to see any studies supporting that claim. Plus, in the clinical trials using 45 mg/day of MK4, the only other nutrients used in some of the studies were calcium and vitamin D3. They had no other ingredients. Magnesium simply was not required to get the incredible fracture reductions seen in the studies.

Don't get me wrong. I'm a huge fan of magnesium. It's estimated that 56% of people don't get enough magnesium in their diets.[79] Therefore, taking a multivitamin and mineral supplement that contains magnesium is a good idea for most people. But the research doesn't support including magnesium in a bone health supplement.

## Omega-3 Fatty Acids

Omega-3 fatty acids are polyunsaturated fatty acids that have anti-inflammatory actions and lots of research showing cardiovascular benefits. In fact, a 2017 review of the research by the American Heart Association (AHA) concluded that omega-3 fatty acids may be helpful supporting heart health.[80] Studies have also shown omega-3 fatty acids promote healthy mood, blood pressure and inflammation balance.[81]

However, there are no studies showing omega-3 fatty acids maintain bone strength. Some bone-building supplements contain omega-3 fatty acids, but in much lower doses than those recommended for heart health and health in other areas of the body. While theoretically plausible, there are no studies showing that omega-3 fatty acids support healthy bone density or reduce fractures.

## Soy Isoflavones

Soy isoflavones refers to multiple naturally occurring chemicals called phytoestrogens. As the name implies, these molecules have estrogenic activity. Since estrogen supplementation has been approved by the FDA as an osteoporosis treatment approach, soy isoflavones have been studied for their bone building effects. Observational studies and clinical trials have not shown any consistent evidence that soy isoflavones can build stronger bones.

## ♫ Take Action ♫

If you take a bone health dietary supplement, grab the bottle now. Compare the ingredients listed in the product's Supplement Facts Panel with those in this chapter.

For bone health, my approach is to keep it simple. Take nutrients shown to reduce fractures; however, since strontium can create some health risks, cause false bone density test results and may interfere with calcium absorption, you're best to avoid it.

The most targeted nutrients for bone health are MK4 (45 mg/day), calcium and vitamin D3. Those nutrients have been shown to promote healthy bone density, reduce fractures and have excellent safety profiles. The dietary supplements, Osteo-K and Osteo-K Minis, that I created for my patients contain these nutrients in the doses used in clinical trials. I formulated them in 2006 when I couldn't find what I needed to help my patients.

In addition, collagen is an important nutrient for maintaining strong bones. While collagen hasn't been shown in clinical trials to reduce fractures, the fact that we know its importance for bone strength, that it was shown to promote faster bone healing and that it promotes healthy bone metabolism, I suggest people also take collagen.

For more information about dietary supplements, go to nbihealth.com.

# Chapter 12

# Social Support

Social support might seem like an odd topic to have in a book about bone health. I've never heard it mentioned at medical conferences. Other healthcare professionals have never discussed this with my patients. But in a medical system that incentivizes writing prescriptions and doing procedures over the "softer science" of health promotion, the research is clear. Your bones—and you—depend on others.

**Your bones—and you—depend on others.**

Feeling connected to others is one of those non-negotiables of health like food and water. Social support nourishes our emotional brains, can give us purpose for working to improve our health, can catch us when we're down and help build us back up.

The research is clear. Having a healthy social support network is associated with a lower osteoporosis risk. When thinking about this, researchers wondered if it's the size or the quality of the relationships that matter. It turns out that they're both important. Yes, size matters, but only to a

**The research is clear. Having a healthy social support network is associated with a lower osteoporosis risk.**

point. In one study, having a strong social support network with three (not four, five or six) other people was associated with the lowest risk of osteoporosis.[1] In other studies, good friends or a supportive partner have been shown to help by providing financial aid or useful information, emotional support, stress reduction and by lowering inflammation and inspiring us to improve our diet and exercise.[2-6] I know my wife and I are both better and healthier because we encourage and push each other to eat healthy, exercise and take care of ourselves. And we have good friends who also help build us up and inspire us to do better and be better. They tell us we also do the same for them.

But just having friends isn't enough. You've got to do stuff with them. Researchers found that the more people interacted with friends and relatives and participated in social activities, the lower their risk for dying compared to people who were more isolated. Those who were living with their significant other also fared better. The highest social interaction scores were associated with a 30% lower risk of dying from any cause. They also had lower risks of dying from heart disease, stroke, diabetes and Alzheimer's.[7] While the study didn't specifically look at death from osteoporosis, a 30% drop in death from any cause includes osteoporosis. Other research concluded that poor social support is associated with a faster loss of hip BMD and worse recovery from hip fractures.[8,9]

While a lot of people may have a great social support system and connections, there are a bunch of folks who don't. A 2012 study determined that among Americans 65 years old and older, which is the highest risk category for osteoporosis, 43% rated themselves as feeling left out, isolated and lacking companionship. In a word, they felt lonely.[10] Loneliness was associated with poor outcomes on all measures. Lonely people were more likely to experience a decreased ability to take care of their basic daily needs like feeding, dressing, going to the bathroom by themselves and bathing; develop problems with completing upper extremity tasks (eg, extending their arms over their shoulders, carrying weights more than 10 pounds); decreased mobility (eg, walking or jogging); and difficulty climbing stairs.

Since COVID, even more people are feeling isolated and alone.[11] If you have family and friends you can connect with, then the answer is straightforward. Reach out to them. Put in the effort. But if you don't have a network you can reach out to, there's one thing you (and everyone) can do—volunteer.

## Volunteer to Connect

Being kind to others is a common teaching in all religions. Christianity, Judaism, Islam, Hinduism and Buddhism all emphasize the importance of doing acts of loving kindness. It seems that science has caught up with what religions and societies have known for thousands of years—being good to others is good for us.

> Science has caught up with what religions and societies have known for thousands of years—being good to others is good for us.

Scientists have shown that kindness not only counteracts stress and depression, it's also associated with improved physical health. Researchers at the University of Massachusetts studied a group of middle-aged adults and found that those who volunteered were less likely to have high blood pressure and elevated cholesterol.[12] Being kind and volunteering have also been shown to improve self-esteem and provide meaning, value and purpose to the one doing the good deed.[13]

It's not simply the act of doing something good for someone else that matters, the intention behind the action is also important. Studies have shown that selfless caregivers (meaning the caregiver isn't looking to advance their career, protect themselves or make a show of their kindness), have better health outcomes than those who are motivated by self-interest, such as advancing their career or expanding their social network.[14,15]

Compared to those who were motivated by self-interest, those who volunteered with the more altruistic goal of helping others benefited more. Those who volunteered out of a sense of kindness and generosity had a lower risk for falls, which reduced their fracture risk. They also had a lower risk of dying from any cause, including dying from osteoporosis.

And if that weren't enough to convince you that getting involved is worth it, they also:

• lived longer
• had better mental and physical health
• had greater life satisfaction

- had fewer functional limitations
- had less disability
- had fewer symptoms of depression

Some of the newest studies on the topic show that random acts of kindness appear to be natural painkillers, too.[16-18]

When you focus on what you can give instead of what you can get, the research is clear. Not only does it reduce pain, but it improves mood, increases your life satisfaction and reduces your risk for heart disease, falling, disability and dying early. There's a lot of need in our communities. Pick something you love and take that passion and use it to help others. You'll feel better and be better for it.

## ♫ Take Action ♫

Like the African proverb says, "If you want to go fast, go alone; but if you want to go far, go together."

This means that you need to find your people. If you've already got a strong network that supports you and builds you up, then fantastic! If you don't, work toward finding even just one or two people who can support you. But it's not a one-way street. You should also build them up and help them too. That's why I recommend people find a workout partner, or someone who they can cook with or do other healthy activities together.

**Do you feel like you have fantastic social support?**

_____

**Are you feeling isolated because you don't have enough people in your life, or that the people in your life aren't the right ones for the support you need now?**

_____

If you've got people in your life, but they're not building you up and supporting you in ways you need, deal with it. Remember what I wrote in Chapter 9 about dealing with problems and not letting them fester? Well now's your chance to do that. Tell people what you need from them and how you'd like to be treated. And if they can't do that for you, find others who can.

If you're socially isolated or simply want to connect with more people, join a club or volunteer.

**Which activities would be fun and meaningful for you to do that could also increase the number of people you meet?**

_____

_____

_____

_____

Whatever you wrote in the blank line, reach out right now and make a plan to get started.

## Chapter 13

# To Your Fracture-Free Future

I know an osteopenia or osteoporosis diagnosis is scary and can be overwhelming. You can feel helpless, and even hopeless. But I hope in these pages you've learned a lot about all the ways you can be in control of this disease, improve your bone health and reduce your fracture risk.

I hope you feel more knowledgeable and equipped to work with your healthcare providers as an active participant instead of simply accepting everything you're told to take. You now have the Take Action blueprint to:

- reduce your risk for falls
- talk to your pharmacist and doctors about medications you're taking that might be damaging your bones and increasing your risk for falls and fractures
- transition into following my Osteoporosis Diet to promote healthier bones and stronger muscles
- safely exercise to improve your strength and balance
- reduce the bone-damaging stress hormone cortisol and live a healthier, more balanced life
- sleep better to improve the health of your bones, body and mind

- choose dietary supplements supported by the research that promote bone health and stronger bones

In the previous chapter on living with purpose, I talked about how helping others helps your own health. If you found solace, solutions, inspiration and a road map to better health in this book, help others by sharing it with your friends and family and on social media. You'll not only help them, but also help me fulfill one of my life missions: educate the public and healthcare providers about how we can all do a better job at reducing the needless pain and suffering caused by osteoporosis.

I hope we keep in touch. I want to hear about your progress and cheer you on in your successes and setbacks. And I want to continue to be a resource for you. You can always find me on Facebook or Twitter, Instagram and LinkedIn under the handle @johnneustadt. And if you just want me in your inbox, you can subscribe to my newsletter at nbihealth.com.

Here's to your health!

*John Neustadt, ND*

Dr. John Neustadt, ND

# References

## Chapter 1

1. Albright F, Smith PH, Richardson AM. Postmenopausal Osteoporosis: Its Clinical Features. *Journal of the American Medical Association.* 1941;116(22):2465-2474.

2. Czerwinski E, Badurski JE, Marcinowska-Suchowierska E, Osieleniec J. Current understanding of osteoporosis according to the position of the World Health Organization (WHO) and International Osteoporosis Foundation. *Ortopedia, traumatologia, rehabilitacja.* 2007;9(4):337-356.

3. Hip Fractures Among Older Adults. Centers for Disease Control and Prevention, National Center for Injury Prevention and Control. https://www.cdc.gov/homeandrecreationalsafety/falls/adulthipfx.html. Published 2016. Accessed April 15, 2021.

4. Abrahamsen B, van Staa T, Ariely R, Olson M, Cooper C. Excess mortality following hip fracture: a systematic epidemiological review. *Osteoporos Int.* 2009;20(10):1633-1650.

5. Bliuc D, Nguyen ND, Milch VE, Nguyen TV, Eisman JA, Center JR. Mortality Risk Associated With Low-Trauma Osteoporotic Fracture and Subsequent Fracture in Men and Women. *JAMA.* 2009;301(5):513-521.

6. Dyer SM, Crotty M, Fairhall N, et al. A critical review of the long-term disability outcomes following hip fracture. *BMC Geriatr.* 2016;16:158.

7. Old JL, Calvert M. Vertebral compression fractures in the elderly. *Am Fam Physician.* 2004;69(1):111-116.

8. Cooper C, Atkinson EJ, Jacobsen SJ, O'Fallon WM, Melton LJ, 3rd. Population-based study of survival after osteoporotic fractures. *Am J Epidemiol.* 1993;137(9):1001-1005.

9. Marshall D, Johnell O, Wedel H. Meta-analysis of how well measures of bone mineral density predict occurrence of osteoporotic fractures. *BMJ.* 1996;312(7041):1254-1259.

10. Liu H, Paige NM, Goldzweig CL. Screening for Osteoporosis in Men: A Systematic Review for an American College of Physicians Guideline. *Ann Intern Med.* 2008;148(9):685-701.

11. Management of osteoporosis in postmenopausal women: 2010 position statement of The North American Menopause Society. *Menopause.* 2010;17(1):25-54.

12. Kanis JA, Johansson H, Harvey NC, McCloskey EV. A brief history of FRAX. *Archives of osteoporosis.* 2018;13(1):118-118.

13. Hoff M, Meyer HE, Skurtveit S, et al. Validation of FRAX and the impact of self-reported falls among elderly in a general population: the HUNT study, Norway. *Osteoporos Int.* 2017;28(10):2935-2944.

14. Salminen H, Piispanen P, Toth-Pal E. Primary care physicians' views on osteoporosis management: a qualitative study. *Arch Osteoporos.* 2019;14(1):48.

15. Curtis JR, Carbone L, Cheng H, et al. Longitudinal trends in use of bone mass measurement among older americans, 1999-2005. *J Bone Miner Res.* 2008;23(7):1061-1067.

16. King AB, Fiorentino DM. Medicare payment cuts for osteoporosis testing reduced use despite tests' benefit in reducing fractures. *Health Aff (Millwood).* 2011;30(12):2362-2370.

17. Lim SY, Lim JH, Nguyen D, et al. Screening for osteoporosis in men aged 70 years and older in a primary care setting in the United States. *Am J Mens Health.* 2013;7(4):350-354.

18. Zhang J, Delzell E, Zhao H, et al. Central DXA utilization shifts from office-based to hospital-based settings among medicare beneficiaries in the wake of reimbursement changes. *J Bone Miner Res.* 2012;27(4):858-864.

19. Oertel MJ, Graves L, Al-Hihi E, et al. Osteoporosis management in older patients who experienced a fracture. *Clinical interventions in aging.* 2016;11:1111-1116.

20. Reducing Falls and Resulting Hip Fractures Among Older Women. Centers for Disease Control and Prevention. Mortality and Morbidicty

Weekly Report (MMWR) Web site. https://www.cdc.gov/mmwr/pre-view/mmwrhtml/rr4902a2.htm. Published March 31, 2000. Accessed April 15, 2021.

21. Shaver AL, Clark CM, Hejna M, Feuerstein S, Wahler RG, Jr., Jacobs DM. Trends in fall-related mortality and fall risk increasing drugs among older individuals in the United States,1999-2017. *Pharmacoepidemiol Drug Saf.* 2021.

## Chapter 2

1. Osteoporosis. National Institutes of Health. https://www.bones.nih.gov/health-info/bone/osteoporosis. Accessed January 14, 2021.

2. Cooper C, Campion G, Melton LJ, 3rd. Hip fractures in the elderly: a world-wide projection. *Osteoporos Int.* 1992;2(6):285-289.

3. *The Burden of Brittle Bones: Epidemiology, Costs & Burden of Osteoporosis in Australia – 2007.* Sydney, Australia: Osteoporosis Australia;2007.

4. Sarafrazi N, Wambogo EA, Shepherd JA. *Osteoporosis or low bone mass in older adults: United States, 2017–2018.* Hyattsville, MD: National Center for Health Statistics;2021.

5. 65 and Older Population Grows Rapidly as Baby Boomers Age. United States Census Bureau. https://www.census.gov/newsroom/press-releases/2020/65-older-population-grows.html. Published June 25, 2020. Accessed October 30, 2020.

6. Ortman JM, Velkoff VA, Hogan H. *An Aging Nation: The Older Population in the United States.* Washington, DC: US Census Bureau;2014.

7. Dennison E, Mohamed MA, Cooper C. Epidemiology of osteoporosis. *Rheumatic diseases clinics of North America.* 2006;32(4):617-629.

8. The Global Burden of Osteoporosis: A Fact Sheet. https://www.iofbonehealth.org/sites/default/files/media/PDFs/Fact%20Sheets/2014-factsheet-osteoporosis-A4.pdf. Accessed August 9, 2017. Accessed August 9, 2017.

9. Kanis JA. Assessment of osteoporosis at the primary health-care level. Technical Report. World Health Organization Collaborating Centre for Metabolic Bone Diseases. University of Sheffiled, UK. https://www.iofbonehealth.org/sites/default/files/WHO_Technical_Report-2007.pdf. Published 2007. Accessed October 14, 2020.

10. Osteoporosis Fast Facts. National Osteoporosis Foundation. . https://cdn.nof.org/wp-content/uploads/2015/12/Osteoporosis-Fast-Facts.pdf. Published 2020. Accessed October 14, 2020.

11. Kanis JA, Delmas P, Burckhardt P, Cooper C, Torgerson D. Guidelines for diagnosis and management of osteoporosis. The European Foundation for Osteoporosis and Bone Disease. *Osteoporos Int.* 1997;7(4):390-406.

12. Cheng S, Levy A, Lefaivre K, Guy P, Kuramoto L, Sobolev B. Geographic trends in incidence of hip fractures: a comprehensive literature review. *Osteoporosis International.* 2011;22(10):2575-2586.

13. United Nations Population Fund (UNFPA) Asia and the Pacific (2020) Ageing. . UNFPA https://asiapacific.unfpa.org/en/node/15208. Accessed January 2, 2022.

14. Lau EM. Osteoporosis--a worldwide problem and the implications in Asia. *Ann Acad Med Singapore.* 2002;31(1):67-68.

15. Riggs BL, Melton I, L. J. The worldwide problem of osteoporosis: Insights afforded by epidemiology. *Bone.* 1995;17(5, Supplement 1):S505-S511.

16. *The Asian Audit: Epidemiology, costs and burden of osteoporosis in Asia 2009.* Switzerland: International Osteoporosis Foundation;2009.

17. Mithal A, Bansal B, Kyer CS, Ebeling P. The Asia-Pacific Regional Audit-Epidemiology, Costs, and Burden of Osteoporosis in India 2013: A report of International Osteoporosis Foundation. *Indian journal of endocrinology and metabolism.* 2014;18(4):449-454.

18. Wang L, Yu W, Yin X, et al. Prevalence of Osteoporosis and Fracture in China: The China Osteoporosis Prevalence Study. *JAMA Network Open.* 2021;4(8):e2121106-e2121106.

19. Cui L, Chen L, Xia W, et al. Vertebral fracture in postmenopausal Chinese women: a population-based study. *Osteoporos Int.* 2017;28(9):2583-2590.

20. Saigal R, Mathur V, Prashant R, Chakraborty A, Mittal V. Glucocorticoid-induced osteoporosis. *Indian Journal of Rheumatology.* 2006;1:20-25.

21. Kanis JA, Norton N, Harvey NC, et al. SCOPE 2021: a new scorecard for osteoporosis in Europe. *Archives of Osteoporosis.* 2021;16(1):82.

22. Kanis JA, Johnell O. Requirements for DXA for the management of osteoporosis in Europe. *Osteoporos Int.* 2005;16(3):229-238.

23. Borgström F, Karlsson L, Ortsäter G, et al. Fragility fractures in Europe: burden, management and opportunities. *Archives of Osteoporosis.* 2020;15(1):59-59.

24. Rodrigues AM, Canhao H, Marques A, et al. Portuguese recommendations for the prevention, diagnosis and management of primary osteoporosis - 2018 update. *Acta Reumatol Port.* Jan-Mar 2018;43(1):10-31.

25. Marques A, Lourenço Ó, da Silva JA. The burden of osteoporotic hip fractures in Portugal: costs, health related quality of life and mortality. *Osteoporos Int.* Nov 2015;26(11):2623-30.

26. Maalouf G, Gannagé-Yared MH, Ezzedine J, et al. Middle East and North Africa consensus on osteoporosis. *J Musculoskelet Neuronal Interact.* 2007;7(2):131-143.

27. El Maghraoui A, Morjane F, Nouijai A, Achemlal L, Bezza A, Ghozlani I. Vertebral fracture assessment in Moroccan women: prevalence and risk factors. *Maturitas.* 2009;62(2):171-175.

28. Cankurtaran M, Yavuz BB, Halil M, Dagli N, Ariogul S. General characteristics, clinical features and related factors of osteoporosis in a group of elderly Turkish men. *Aging clinical and experimental research.* 2005;17(2):108-115.

## Chapter 3

1. Lu J, Shin Y, Yen MS, Sun SS. Peak Bone Mass and Patterns of Change in Total Bone Mineral Density and Bone Mineral Contents From Childhood Into Young Adulthood. *J Clin Densitom.* 2016;19(2):180-191.

2. McGarry KA, Kiel DP. Postmenopausal osteoporosis. Strategies for preventing bone loss, avoiding fracture. *Postgrad Med.* 2000;108(3):79-82, 85-78, 91.

3. Sunyer T, Lewis J, Collin-Osdoby P, Osdoby P. Estrogen's bone-protective effects may involve differential IL-1 receptor regulation in human osteoclast-like cells. *J Clin Invest.* 1999;103(10):1409-1418.

4. Buehler MJ, Yung YC. Deformation and failure of protein materials in physiologically extreme conditions and disease. *Nat Mater.* 2009;8(3):175-188.

5. Burla F, Dussi S, Martinez-Torres C, Tauber J, van der Gucht J, Koenderink GH. Connectivity and plasticity determine collagen network fracture. *Proc Natl Acad Sci U S A.* 2020;117(15):8326-8334.

6. Boskey AL, Wright TM, Blank RD. Collagen and bone strength. *J Bone Miner Res.* 1999;14(3):330-335.

7. Wang X, Bank RA, TeKoppele JM, Hubbard GB, Athanasiou KA, Agrawal CM. Effect of collagen denaturation on the toughness of bone. *Clinical orthopaedics and related research.* 2000(371):228-239.

8. Zioupos P, Currey JD, Hamer AJ. The role of collagen in the declining mechanical properties of aging human cortical bone. *Journal of biomedical materials research.* 1999;45(2):108-116.

9. Wadhwa R, Kumar M, Talegaonkar S, Vohora D. Serotonin reuptake inhibitors and bone health: A review of clinical studies and plausible mechanisms. *Osteoporosis and Sarcopenia.* 2017;3(2):75-81.

10. Li T, Jiang S, Lu C, et al. Melatonin: Another avenue for treating osteoporosis? *J Pineal Res.* 2019;66(2):e12548.

11. Guntur AR, Rosen CJ. Bone as an endocrine organ. *Endocr Pract.* 2012;18(5):758-762.

12. Karsenty G, Oury F. Regulation of male fertility by the bone-derived hormone osteocalcin. *Mol Cell Endocrinol.* 2014;382(1):521-526.

13. Berger JM, Singh P, Khrimian L, et al. Mediation of the Acute Stress Response by the Skeleton. *Cell Metab.* 2019;30(5):890-902 e898.

## Chapter 4

1. Schnell S, Friedman SM, Mendelson DA, Bingham KW, Kates SL. The 1-year mortality of patients treated in a hip fracture program for elders. *Geriatr Orthop Surg Rehabil.* 2010;1(1):6-14.

2. Glade MJ. Food, nutrition, and the prevention of cancer: a global perspective. American Institute for Cancer Research/World Cancer Research Fund, American Institute for Cancer Research, 1997. *Nutrition.* 1999;15(6):523-526.

3. *U.S. Department of Health and Human Services. Healthy People 2010: Understanding and Improving Health.* 2d ed. Washington, D.C.: U.S. Government Printing Office; 2000.

4. Fonseca AL, Koyama J, Butler EA. The Role of Family of Origin in Current Lifestyle Choices: A Qualitative Secondary Data Analysis of Interracial and Same-Race Couples. *Family & community health.* 2018;41(3):146-158.

5. Małachowska A, Jeżewska-Zychowicz M. Does Examining the Childhood Food Experiences Help to Better Understand Food Choices in Adulthood? *Nutrients.* 2021;13(3):983.

6. Garriguet D, Colley R, Bushnik T. Parent-Child association in physical activity and sedentary behaviour. *Health Rep.* 2017;28(6):3-11.

7. Sivertsen B, Lallukka T, Salo P, et al. Insomnia as a risk factor for ill health: results from the large population-based prospective HUNT Study in Norway. *J Sleep Res.* 2014;23(2):124-132.

8. Management of osteoporosis in postmenopausal women: 2006 position statement of The North American Menopause Society. *Menopause.* 2006;13(3):340-367; quiz 368-349.

## Chapter 5

1. Brooks M. *US prescriptions hit new high in 2018, but opioid scripts dip.* Medscape Medical News; May 2019.

2. *Therapeutic Drug Use.* Washington, DC: Centers for Disease Control and Prevention; April 2020.

3. Hales CM, Servais J, Martin CB, Kohen D. Prescription Drug Use Among Adults Aged 40-79 in the United States and Canada. *NCHS Data Brief.* 2019(347):1-8.

4. Woodruff K. Preventing polypharmacy in older adults. American Nurse Association. https://www.myamericannurse.com/preventing-polypharmacy-in-older-adults/. Published 2010. Accessed January 18, 2021.

5. Jokanovic N, Tan EC, Dooley MJ, Kirkpatrick CM, Bell JS. Prevalence and factors associated with polypharmacy in long-term care facilities: a systematic review. *J Am Med Dir Assoc.* 2015;16(6):535.e531-512.

6. Safer DJ. Overprescribed Medications for US Adults: Four Major Examples. *J Clin Med Res.* 2019;11(9):617-622.

7. Panday K, Gona A, Humphrey MB. Medication-induced osteoporosis: screening and treatment strategies. *Ther Adv Musculoskelet Dis.* 2014;6(5):185-202.

8. Fitzpatrick LA. Secondary causes of osteoporosis. *Mayo Clin Proc.* 2002;77(5):453-468.

9. Cohen A, Fleischer J, Freeby MJ, McMahon DJ, Irani D, Shane E. Clinical characteristics and medication use among premenopausal women with osteoporosis and low BMD: the experience of an osteoporosis referral center. *J Womens Health (Larchmt).* 2009;18(1):79-84.

10. Ebeling PR. Clinical practice. Osteoporosis in men. *N Engl J Med.* 2008;358(14):1474-1482.

11. Cerdá Gabaroi D, Peris P, Monegal A, et al. Search for hidden secondary causes in postmenopausal women with osteoporosis. *Menopause.* 2010;17(1):135-139.

12. Zaninotto P, Huang YT, Di Gessa G, Abell J, Lassale C, Steptoe A. Polypharmacy is a risk factor for hospital admission due to a fall:

evidence from the English Longitudinal Study of Ageing. *BMC Public Health.* 2020;20(1):1804.

13. Shaver AL, Clark CM, Hejna M, Feuerstein S, Wahler RG, Jr., Jacobs DM. Trends in fall-related mortality and fall risk increasing drugs among older individuals in the United States,1999-2017. *Pharmacoepidemiol Drug Saf.* 2021.

14. Munson JC, Bynum JPW, Bell J-E, et al. Patterns of Prescription Drug Use Before and After Fragility Fracture. *JAMA Internal Medicine.* 2016;176(10):1531-1538.

15. Clark CM, Shaver AL, Aurelio LA, et al. Potentially Inappropriate Medications Are Associated with Increased Healthcare Utilization and Costs. *J Am Geriatr Soc.* 2020;68(11):2542-2550.

16. Compston J. Glucocorticoid-induced osteoporosis: an update. *Endocrine.* 2018;61(1):7-16.

17. Díez-Pérez A, Hooven FH, Adachi JD, et al. Regional differences in treatment for osteoporosis. The Global Longitudinal Study of Osteoporosis in Women (GLOW). *Bone.* 2011;49(3):493-498.

18. Silverman S, Curtis J, Saag K, et al. International management of bone health in glucocorticoid-exposed individuals in the observational GLOW study. *Osteoporos Int.* 2015;26(1):419-420.

19. Canalis E, Mazziotti G, Giustina A, Bilezikian JP. Glucocorticoid-induced osteoporosis: pathophysiology and therapy. *Osteoporos Int.* 2007;18(10):1319-1328.

20. Van Staa TP, Leufkens HGM, Abenhaim L, Zhang B, Cooper C. Use of oral corticosteroids and risk of fractures. *J Bone Miner Res.* 2000;15(6):993-1000.

21. Van Staa TP, Laan RF, Barton IP, Cohen S, Reid DM, Cooper C. Bone density threshold and other predictors of vertebral fracture in patients receiving oral glucocorticoid therapy. *Arthritis Rheum.* 2003;48(11):3224-3229.

22. Chalitsios CV, Shaw DE, McKeever TM. A retrospective database study of oral corticosteroid and bisphosphonate prescribing patterns in England. *NPJ Prim Care Respir Med.* 2020;30(1):5.

23. De Vries F, Bracke M, Leufkens HG, Lammers JW, Cooper C, Van Staa TP. Fracture risk with intermittent high-dose oral glucocorticoid therapy. *Arthritis Rheum.* 2007;56(1):208-214.

24. van Staa TP, Leufkens HG, Abenhaim L, Zhang B, Cooper C. Oral corticosteroids and fracture risk: relationship to daily and cumulative doses. *Rheumatology (Oxford).* 2000;39(12):1383-1389.

25. van Staa TP, Leufkens HG, Cooper C. The epidemiology of corticosteroid-induced osteoporosis: a meta-analysis. *Osteoporos Int.* 2002;13(10):777-787.

26. Nehra AK, Alexander JA, Loftus CG, Nehra V. Proton Pump Inhibitors: Review of Emerging Concerns. *Mayo Clin Proc.* 2018;93(2):240-246.

27. Burlington M. *Declining Medicine Use and Costs: For Better or Worse? A Review of the Use of Medicines in the United States in 2012.* Danbury, CT: IMS Institute for Healthcare Informatics;2013.

28. Chan A, Liang L, Tung ACH, Kinkade A, Tejani AM. Is There a Reason for the Proton Pump Inhibitor? An Assessment of Prescribing for Residential Care Patients in British Columbia. *Can J Hosp Pharm.* 2018;71(5):295-301.

29. FDA Drug Safety Communication: Possible increased risk of fractures of the hip, wrist, and spine with the use of proton pump inhibitors. US Food and Drug Administration. https://www.fda.gov/drugs/postmarket-drug-safety-information-patients-and-providers/fda-drug-safety-communication-possible-increased-risk-fractures-hip-wrist-and-spine-use-proton-pump. Published 2010. Accessed January 19, 2021.

30. Yang YX, Lewis JD, Epstein S, Metz DC. Long-term proton pump inhibitor therapy and risk of hip fracture. *JAMA.* 2006;296(24):2947-2953.

31. Lapumnuaypol K, Thongprayoon C, Wijarnpreecha K, Tiu A, Cheungpasitporn W. Risk of fall in patients taking proton pump inhibitors: a meta-analysis. *QJM: An International Journal of Medicine.* 2019;112(2):115-121.

32. Yang SD, Chen Q, Wei HK, et al. Bone fracture and the interaction between bisphosphonates and proton pump inhibitors: a meta-analysis. *Int J Clin Exp Med.* 2015;8(4):4899-4910.

33. Qorraj-Bytyqi H, Hoxha R, Sadiku S, et al. Proton Pump Inhibitors Intake and Iron and Vitamin B12 Status: A Prospective Comparative Study with a Follow up of 12 Months. *Open Access Maced J Med Sci.* 2018;6(3):442-446.

34. Lúquez Mindiola AJ, Marulanda Fernández H, Rodríguez Arciniegas DE, Otero Regino W. Vitamin B12 Deficiency Associated with Consumption of Proton Pump Inhibitors. *Revista colombiana de Gastroenterología.* 2017;32(3):197-201.

35. Baird-Gunning J, Bromley J. Correcting iron deficiency. *Aust Prescr.* 2016;39(6):193-199.

36. Namaste SM, Rohner F, Huang J, et al. Adjusting ferritin concentrations for inflammation: Biomarkers Reflecting Inflammation and Nutritional Determinants of Anemia (BRINDA) project. *Am J Clin Nutr.* 2017;106(Suppl 1):359S-371S.

37. Goddard AF, James MW, McIntyre AS, Scott BB, British Society of G. Guidelines for the management of iron deficiency anaemia. *Gut.* 2011;60(10):1309-1316.

38. Wang W, Knovich MA, Coffman LG, Torti FM, Torti SV. Serum ferritin: Past, present and future. *Biochim Biophys Acta.* 2010;1800(8):760-769.

39. Kratz A, Ferraro M, Sluss PM, Lewandrowski KB. Case records of the Massachusetts General Hospital. Weekly clinicopathological exercises. Laboratory reference values. *N Engl J Med.* 2004;351(15):1548-1563.

40. Vaucher P, Druais PL, Waldvogel S, Favrat B. Effect of iron supplementation on fatigue in nonanemic menstruating women with low ferritin: a randomized controlled trial. *CMAJ.* 2012;184(11):1247-1254.

41. Mackie S, Winkelman JW. Normal ferritin in a patient with iron deficiency and RLS. *J Clin Sleep Med.* 2013;9(5):511-513.

42. DJ B, Q G. *Antidepressant use among adults: United States, 2015–2018. NCHS Data Brief, no 377.* Hyattsville, MD: National Center for Health Statistics;2020.

43. Moura C, Bernatsky S, Abrahamowicz M, et al. Antidepressant use and 10-year incident fracture risk: the population-based Canadian Multi-centre Osteoporosis Study (CaMoS). *Osteoporos Int.* 2014;25(5):1473-1481.

44. Diem SJ, Blackwell TL, Stone KL, et al. Use of antidepressants and rates of hip bone loss in older women: the study of osteoporotic fractures. *Arch Intern Med.* 2007;167(12):1240-1245.

45. Eom CS, Lee HK, Ye S, Park SM, Cho KH. Use of selective serotonin reuptake inhibitors and risk of fracture: a systematic review and meta-analysis. *J Bone Miner Res.* 2012;27(5):1186-1195.

46. Khanassov V, Hu J, Reeves D, van Marwijk H. Selective serotonin reuptake inhibitor and selective serotonin and norepinephrine reuptake inhibitor use and risk of fractures in adults: A systematic review and meta-analysis. *Int J Geriatr Psychiatry.* 2018;33(12):1688-1708.

47. Carey B, Gebeloff R. Many People Taking Antidepressants Discover They Cannot Quit. *New York Times.* 2018. https://www.nytimes.com/2018/04/07/health/antidepressants-withdrawal-prozac-cymbalta.html. Published April 7, 2018. Accessed April 20, 2021.

48. Penninx BWJH, Guralnik JM, Ferrucci L, Fried LP, Allen RH, Stabler SP. Vitamin B12 Deficiency and Depression in Physically Disabled Older Women: Epidemiologic Evidence From the Women's Health and Aging Study. *Am J Psychiatry.* 2000;157(5):715-721.

49. Merete C, Falcon LM, Tucker KL. Vitamin B6 Is Associated with Depressive Symptomatology in Massachusetts Elders. *J Am Coll Nutr.* 2008;27(3):421-427.

50. Paul RT, McDonnell AP, Kelly CB. Folic acid: neurochemistry, metabolism and relationship to depression. *Hum Psychopharmacol.* 2004;19(7):477-488.

51. Vahdat Shariatpanaahi M, Vahdat Shariatpanaahi Z, Moshtaaghi M, Shahbaazi SH, Abadi A. The relationship between depression and serum ferritin level. *Eur J Clin Nutr.* 2006;61(4):532-535.

52. Booij L, van der Does AJW, Haffmans PMJ, Spinhoven P, McNally RJ. Acute tryptophan depletion as a model of depressive relapse: Behavioural specificity and ethical considerations. *Br J Psychiatry.* 2005;187(2):148-154.

53. Booij L, Van der Does AJW, Haffmans PMJ, Riedel WJ, Fekkes D, Blom MJB. The effects of high-dose and low-dose tryptophan depletion on mood and cognitive functions of remitted depressed patients. *J Psychopharmacol.* 2005;19(3):267-275.

54. Lakhan SE, Vieira KF. Nutritional therapies for mental disorders. *Nutr J.* 2008;7:2.

55. Neustadt J, Pieczenik S. *Foundations and Applications of Medical Biochemistry in Clinical Practice.* iUniverse; 2009.

56. Chen Z, Maricic M, Pettinger M, et al. Osteoporosis and rate of bone loss among postmenopausal survivors of breast cancer. *Cancer.* 2005;104(7):1520-1530.

57. Lindsey AM, Gross G, Twiss J, Waltman N, Ott C, Moore TE. Postmenopausal survivors of breast cancer at risk for osteoporosis: nutritional intake and body size. *Cancer Nurs.* 2002;25(1):50-56.

58. Colzani E, Clements M, Johansson AL, et al. Risk of hospitalisation and death due to bone fractures after breast cancer: a registry-based cohort study. *Br J Cancer.* 2016;115(11):1400-1407.

59. Fabian CJ. The what, why and how of aromatase inhibitors: hormonal agents for treatment and prevention of breast cancer. *Int J Clin Pract.* 2007;61(12):2051-2063.

60. Goldhirsch A, Ingle JN, Gelber RD, Coates AS, Thürlimann B, Senn HJ. Thresholds for therapies: highlights of the St Gallen International Expert Consensus on the primary therapy of early breast cancer 2009. *Ann Oncol.* 2009;20(8):1319-1329.

61. Hadji P, Aapro MS, Body JJ, et al. Management of Aromatase Inhibitor-Associated Bone Loss (AIBL) in postmenopausal women with hormone sensitive breast cancer: Joint position statement of the IOF, CABS, ECTS, IEG, ESCEO IMS, and SIOG. *J Bone Oncol.* 2017;7:1-12.

62. Weitzmann MN, Pacifici R. T cells: unexpected players in the bone loss induced by estrogen deficiency and in basal bone homeostasis. *Ann N Y Acad Sci.* 2007;1116:360-375.

63. Charlson J, Smith EC, Smallwood AJ, Laud PW, Neuner JM. Bone Mineral Density Testing Disparities Among Patients With Breast Cancer Prescribed Aromatase Inhibitors. *J Natl Compr Canc Netw.* 2016;14(7):875-880.

64. Ligibel JA, O'Malley AJ, Fisher M, Daniel GW, Winer EP, Keating NL. Patterns of bone density evaluation in a community population treated with aromatase inhibitors. *Breast Cancer Res Treat.* 2012;134(3):1305-1313.

65. Theriault R, Carlson R, Allred C, et al. National Comprehensive Cancer Network. Breast Cancer, Version 3.2013: Featured Updates to the NCCN Guidelines. *J Natl Compr Canc Netw.* 2013;11(7):753-760.

66. Stratton J, Hu X, Soulos PR, et al. Bone density screening in postmenopausal women with early-stage breast cancer treated with aromatase inhibitors. *Journal of oncology practice.* 2017;13(5):e505-e515.

67. Hillner BE, Ingle JN, Chlebowski RT, et al. American Society of Clinical Oncology 2003 update on the role of bisphosphonates and bone health issues in women with breast cancer. *Journal of Clinical Oncology.* 2003;21(21):4042-4057.

68. Parker WH, Jacoby V, Shoupe D, Rocca W. Effect of Bilateral Oophorectomy on Women's Long-Term Health. *Women's Health.* 2009;5(5):565-576.

69. Bellido T, Jilka RL, Boyce BF, et al. Regulation of interleukin-6, osteoclastogenesis, and bone mass by androgens. The role of the androgen receptor. *J Clin Invest.* 1995;95(6):2886-2895.

70. Kim TJ, Koo KC. Pathophysiology of Bone Loss in Patients with Prostate Cancer Receiving Androgen-Deprivation Therapy and Lifestyle Modifications for the Management of Bone Health: A Comprehensive Review. *Cancers (Basel)*. 2020;12(6).

71. Waibel-Treber S, Minne HW, Scharla SH, Bremen T, Ziegler R, Leyendecker G. Reversible bone loss in women treated with GnRH-agonists for endometriosis and uterine leiomyoma. *Hum Reprod.* 1989;4(4):384-388.

72. Lee CE, Leslie WD, Czaykowski P, Gingerich J, Geirnaert M, Lau YK. A comprehensive bone-health management approach for men with prostate cancer receiving androgen deprivation therapy. *Curr Oncol.* 2011;18(4):e163-172.

73. Hamilton EJ, Ghasem-Zadeh A, Gianatti E, et al. Structural decay of bone microarchitecture in men with prostate cancer treated with androgen deprivation therapy. *J Clin Endocrinol Metab.* 2010;95(12):E456-463.

74. Morote J, Morin JP, Orsola A, et al. Prevalence of osteoporosis during long-term androgen deprivation therapy in patients with prostate cancer. *Urology.* 2007;69(3):500-504.

75. Smith MR, Lee WC, Brandman J, Wang Q, Botteman M, Pashos CL. Gonadotropin-Releasing Hormone Agonists and Fracture Risk: A Claims-Based Cohort Study of Men With Nonmetastatic Prostate Cancer. *Journal of Clinical Oncology.* 2005;23(31):7897-7903.

76. Shahinian VB, Kuo Y-F, Freeman JL, Goodwin JS. Risk of Fracture after Androgen Deprivation for Prostate Cancer. *New England Journal of Medicine.* 2005;352(2):154-164.

77. Brown J, Pan A, Hart RJ. Gonadotrophin-releasing hormone analogues for pain associated with endometriosis. *Cochrane Database Syst Rev.* 2010;2010(12):Cd008475.

78. Saylor PJ, Keating NL, Smith MR. Prostate cancer survivorship: prevention and treatment of the adverse effects of androgen deprivation therapy. *J Gen Intern Med.* 2009;24 Suppl 2(Suppl 2):S389-394.

79. Somekawa Y, Chigughi M, Harada M, Ishibashi T. Use of vitamin K2 (menatetrenone) and 1,25-dihydroxyvitamin D3 in the prevention of bone loss induced by leuprolide. *J Clin Endocrinol Metab.* 1999;84(8):2700-2704.

## Chapter 6

1. Fitzpatrick LA. Secondary causes of osteoporosis. *Mayo Clin Proc.* 2002;77(5):453-468.

2. Cohen A, Fleischer J, Freeby MJ, McMahon DJ, Irani D, Shane E. Clinical characteristics and medication use among premenopausal women with osteoporosis and low BMD: the experience of an osteoporosis referral center. *J Womens Health (Larchmt).* 2009;18(1):79-84.

3. Ebeling PR. Clinical practice. Osteoporosis in men. *N Engl J Med.* 2008;358(14):1474-1482.

4. Cerdá Gabaroi D, Peris P, Monegal A, et al. Search for hidden secondary causes in postmenopausal women with osteoporosis. *Menopause.* 2010;17(1):135-139.

5. Balasubramanian A, Zhang J, Chen L, et al. Risk of subsequent fracture after prior fracture among older women. *Osteoporos Int.* 2019;30(1):79-92.

6. Burge R, Dawson-Hughes B, Solomon DH, Wong JB, King A, Tosteson A. Incidence and Economic Burden of Osteoporosis-Related Fractures in the United States, 2005-2025. *Journal of Bone and Mineral Research.* 2007;22(3):465-475.

7. Tsuda T, Hashimoto Y, Okamoto Y, Ando W, Ebina K. Meta-analysis for the efficacy of bisphosphonates on hip fracture prevention. *Journal of Bone and Mineral Metabolism.* 2020;38(5):678-686.

8. Wen F, Du H, Ding L, et al. Clinical efficacy and safety of drug interventions for primary and secondary prevention of osteoporotic fractures in postmenopausal women: Network meta-analysis followed by factor and cluster analysis. *PLoS One.* 2020;15(6):e0234123.

9. Muñoz-Torres M, Alonso G, Raya MP. Calcitonin therapy in osteoporosis. *Treat Endocrinol.* 2004;3(2):117-132.

10. Shi L, Min N, Wang F, Xue Q-Y. Bisphosphonates for Secondary Prevention of Osteoporotic Fractures: A Bayesian Network Meta-Analysis of Randomized Controlled Trials. *BioMed Research International.* 2019;2019:2594149.

11. Lyles KW, Colon-Emeric CS, Magaziner JS, et al. Zoledronic acid and clinical fractures and mortality after hip fracture. *N Engl J Med.* 2007;357(18):1799-1809.

12. Girgis CM, Sher D, Seibel MJ. Atypical femoral fractures and bisphosphonate use. *N Engl J Med.* 2010;362(19):1848-1849.

13. Compston J. Pathophysiology of atypical femoral fractures and osteonecrosis of the jaw. *Osteoporosis International.* 2011;22(12):2951-2961.

14. Schilcher J, Koeppen V, Aspenberg P, Michaëlsson K. Risk of atypical femoral fracture during and after bisphosphonate use. *Acta Orthop.* 2015;86(1):100-107.

15. Sedghizadeh PP, Stanley K, Caligiuri M, Hofkes S, Lowry B, Shuler CF. Oral bisphosphonate use and the prevalence of osteonecrosis of the jaw: An institutional inquiry. *J Am Dent Assoc.* 2009;140(1):61-66.

16. Otto S, Abu-Id MH, Fedele S, et al. Osteoporosis and bisphosphonates-related osteonecrosis of the jaw: Not just a sporadic coincidence - a multi-centre study. *Journal of Cranio-Maxillofacial Surgery.* 2011;39(4):272-277.

17. Huybrechts KF, Ishak KJ, Caro JJ. Assessment of compliance with osteoporosis treatment and its consequences in a managed care population. *Bone.* 2006;38(6):922-928.

18. Seeman E, Compston J, Adachi J, et al. Non-compliance: the Achilles' heel of anti-fracture efficacy. *Osteoporos Int.* 2007;18(6):711-719.

19. Curtis JR, Westfall AO, Cheng H, Lyles K, Saag KG, Delzell E. Benefit of adherence with bisphosphonates depends on age and fracture type: results from an analysis of 101,038 new bisphosphonate users. *J Bone Miner Res.* 2008;23(9):1435-1441.

## Chapter 7

1. *Average daily intake of nutrients by food source and demographic characteristics, 2015–16 and 2017–18.* US Department of Agriculture Economic Research Service; April 1 2021.

2. Aubry A. The Average American Ate (Literally) A Ton This Year. In. *The Salt: What's on Your Plate*: NPR; 2011.

3. Data, Trend and Maps [online]. Centers for Disease Control Prevention, National Center for Chronic Disease Prevention and Health Promotion, Division of Nutrition, Physical Activity, and Obesity. https://www.cdc.gov/nccdphp/dnpao/data-trends-maps/index.html. Accessed May 10, 2021.

4. Movassagh EZ, Vatanparast H. Current Evidence on the Association of Dietary Patterns and Bone Health: A Scoping Review. *Adv Nutr.* 2017;8(1):1-16.

5. Ilich JZ, Kelly OJ, Kim Y, Spicer MT. Low-grade chronic inflammation perpetuated by modern diet as a promoter of obesity and osteoporosis. *Arh Hig Rada Toksikol.* 2014;65(2):139-148.

6. Reddy MB, Love M. The impact of food processing on the nutritional quality of vitamins and minerals. *Adv Exp Med Biol.* 1999;459:99-106.

7. Agte V, Tarwadi K, Mengale S, Hinge A, Chiplonkar S. Vitamin profile of cooked foods: how healthy is the practice of ready-to-eat foods? *International journal of food sciences and nutrition.* 2002;53(3):197-208.

8. Nesheim RO. Nutrient changes in food processing. A current review. *Fed Proc.* 1974;33(11):2267-2269.

9. Schroeder HA. Losses of vitamins and trace minerals resulting from processing and preservation of foods. *Am J Clin Nutr.* 1971;24(5):562-573.

10. Langsetmo L, Poliquin S, Hanley DA, et al. Dietary patterns in Canadian men and women ages 25 and older: relationship to demographics, body mass index, and bone mineral density. *BMC Musculoskelet Disord.* 2010;11:20.

11. Okubo H, Sasaki S, Horiguchi H, et al. Dietary patterns associated with bone mineral density in premenopausal Japanese farmwomen. *Am J Clin Nutr.* 2006;83(5):1185-1192.

12. Zeng FF, Wu BH, Fan F, et al. Dietary patterns and the risk of hip fractures in elderly Chinese: a matched case-control study. *J Clin Endocrinol Metab.* 2013;98(6):2347-2355.

13. Palomeras-Vilches A, Vinals-Mayolas E, Bou-Mias C, et al. Adherence to the Mediterranean Diet and Bone Fracture Risk in Middle-Aged Women: A Case Control Study. *Nutrients.* 2019;11(10).

14. Samieri C, Ginder Coupez V, Lorrain S, et al. Nutrient patterns and risk of fracture in older subjects: results from the Three-City Study. *Osteoporos Int.* 2013;24(4):1295-1305.

15. Byberg L, Bellavia A, Larsson SC, Orsini N, Wolk A, Michaëlsson K. Mediterranean Diet and Hip Fracture in Swedish Men and Women. *J Bone Miner Res.* 2016;31(12):2098-2105.

16. Haring B, Crandall CJ, Wu C, et al. Dietary Patterns and Fractures in Postmenopausal Women: Results From the Women's Health Initiative. *JAMA Intern Med.* 2016;176(5):645-652.

17. Bliuc D, Nguyen ND, Milch VE, Nguyen TV, Eisman JA, Center JR. Mortality Risk Associated With Low-Trauma Osteoporotic Fracture and Subsequent Fracture in Men and Women. *JAMA.* 2009;301(5):513-521.

18. Sim M, Lewis JR, Blekkenhorst LC, et al. Dietary nitrate intake is associated with muscle function in older women. *J Cachexia Sarcopenia Muscle.* 2019;10(3):601-610.

19. Sim M, Blekkenhorst LC, Bondonno NP, et al. Dietary Nitrate Intake Is Positively Associated with Muscle Function in Men and Women Independent of Physical Activity Levels. *The Journal of Nutrition.* 2021;151(5):1222-1230.

20. Tang X, Ma S, Li Y, et al. Evaluating the Activity of Sodium Butyrate to Prevent Osteoporosis in Rats by Promoting Osteal GSK-3β/Nrf2 Signaling and Mitochondrial Function. *Journal of Agricultural and Food Chemistry.* 2020;68(24):6588-6603.

21. Nutrient density by food source and demographic characteristics, 2015–16 and 2017–18. US Department of Agriculture, Economic Research Service. https://www.ers.usda.gov/data-products/food-consumption-and-nutrient-intakes/. Updated April 1, 2021. Accessed May 10, 2021.

22. Neustadt J. Western Diet and Inflammation. *Integr Med.* 2006;5(4):14-18.

23. Baum JI, Kim IY, Wolfe RR. Protein Consumption and the Elderly: What Is the Optimal Level of Intake? *Nutrients.* 2016;8(6).

24. Roubenoff R, Hughes VA. Sarcopenia: current concepts. *J Gerontol A Biol Sci Med Sci.* 2000;55(12):M716-724.

25. Heymsfield SB, Fearnbach N. Can increasing physical activity prevent aging-related loss of skeletal muscle? *The American Journal of Clinical Nutrition.* 2021.

26. Yu R, Leung J, Woo J. Incremental predictive value of sarcopenia for incident fracture in an elderly Chinese cohort: results from the Osteoporotic Fractures in Men (MrOs) Study. *J Am Med Dir Assoc.* 2014;15(8):551-558.

27. Yoo JI, Kim H, Ha YC, Kwon HB, Koo KH. Osteosarcopenia in Patients with Hip Fracture Is Related with High Mortality. *J Korean Med Sci.* 2018;33(4):e27.

28. Alswat KA. Gender Disparities in Osteoporosis. *Journal of clinical medicine research.* 2017;9(5):382-387.

29. Nowson C, O'Connell S. Protein Requirements and Recommendations for Older People: A Review. *Nutrients.* 2015;7(8):6874-6899.

30. Isanejad M, Sirola J, Mursu J, Kröger H, Tuppurainen M, Erkkilä AT. Association of Protein Intake with Bone Mineral Density and Bone Mineral Content among Elderly Women: The OSTPRE Fracture Prevention Study. *J Nutr Health Aging.* 2017;21(6):622-630.

## Chapter 8

1. Sinaki M, Mikkelsen BA. Postmenopausal spinal osteoporosis: flexion versus extension exercises. *Arch Phys Med Rehabil.* 1984;65(10):593-596.

2. *2018 Participation Report: The Physical Activity Council's annual study tracking sports, fitness, and recreation participation in the US.* Physical Activity Council;2018.

3. Brocklebank LA, Falconer CL, Page AS, Perry R, Cooper AR. Accelerometer-measured sedentary time and cardiometabolic biomarkers: A systematic review. *Prev Med.* 2015;76:92-102.

4. Zhou Y, Zhao H, Peng C. Association of sedentary behavior with the risk of breast cancer in women: update meta-analysis of observational studies. *Ann Epidemiol.* 2015;25(9):687-697.

5. Howe TE, Shea B, Dawson LJ, et al. Exercise for preventing and treating osteoporosis in postmenopausal women. *Cochrane Database Syst Rev.* 2011(7):Cd000333.

6. Zhai L, Zhang Y, Zhang D. Sedentary behaviour and the risk of depression: a meta-analysis. *Br J Sports Med.* 2015;49(11):705-709.

7. Lee J, Chang RW, Ehrlich-Jones L, et al. Sedentary behavior and physical function: objective evidence from the Osteoarthritis Initiative. *Arthritis Care Res (Hoboken).* 2015;67(3):366-373.

8. Steinberg SI, Sammel MD, Harel BT, et al. Exercise, sedentary pastimes, and cognitive performance in healthy older adults. *Am J Alzheimers Dis Other Demen.* 2015;30(3):290-298.

9. de Rezende LF, Rey-López JP, Matsudo VK, do Carmo Luiz O. Sedentary behavior and health outcomes among older adults: a systematic review. *BMC Public Health.* 2014;14:333.

10. Pavey TG, Peeters GG, Brown WJ. Sitting-time and 9-year all-cause mortality in older women. *Br J Sports Med.* 2015;49(2):95-99.

11. Biswas A, Oh PI, Faulkner GE, et al. Sedentary time and its association with risk for disease incidence, mortality, and hospitalization in adults: a systematic review and meta-analysis. *Ann Intern Med.* 2015;162(2):123-132.

12. Moayyeri A. The association between physical activity and osteoporotic fractures: a review of the evidence and implications for future research. *Ann Epidemiol.* 2008;18(11):827-835.

13. Eijsvogels TM, Thompson PD. Exercise Is Medicine: At Any Dose? *Jama*. 2015;314(18):1915-1916.

14. Paluch AE, Gabriel KP, Fulton JE, et al. Steps per Day and All-Cause Mortality in Middle-aged Adults in the Coronary Artery Risk Development in Young Adults Study. *JAMA Network Open*. 2021;4(9):e2124516-e2124516.

15. Saint-Maurice PF, Troiano RP, Bassett DR, Jr., et al. Association of Daily Step Count and Step Intensity With Mortality Among US Adults. *Jama*. 2020;323(12):1151-1160.

16. Lee I-M, Shiroma EJ, Kamada M, Bassett DR, Matthews CE, Buring JE. Association of Step Volume and Intensity With All-Cause Mortality in Older Women. *JAMA Internal Medicine*. 2019;179(8):1105-1112.

17. Crum AJ, Langer EJ. Mind-set matters: exercise and the placebo effect. *Psychol Sci*. 2007;18(2):165-171.

18. Hamer M, Chida Y. Walking and primary prevention: a meta-analysis of prospective cohort studies. *British Journal of Sports Medicine*. 2007;42:238-243.

19. Siddarth D, Siddarth P, Lavretsky H. An observational study of the health benefits of yoga or tai chi compared with aerobic exercise in community-dwelling middle-aged and older adults. *Am J Geriatr Psychiatry*. 2014;22(3):272-273.

20. Abreu M, Hartley G. The effects of Salsa dance on balance, gait, and fall risk in a sedentary patient with Alzheimer's dementia, multiple comorbidities, and recurrent falls. *J Geriatr Phys Ther*. 2013;36(2):100-108.

## Chapter 9

1. *Stress in America: The State of Our Nation. Stress in America Survey.*: American Psychological Association;2017.

2. *Stress in America 2020: A National Mental Health Crisis.* American Psychological Association;2020.

3. Dhabhar FS. Effects of stress on immune function: the good, the bad, and the beautiful. *Immunol Res.* 2014;58(2-3):193-210.

4. Lebedeva A, Sundström A, Lindgren L, et al. Longitudinal relationships among depressive symptoms, cortisol, and brain atrophy in the neocortex and the hippocampus. *Acta Psychiatr Scand.* 2018;137(6):491-502.

5. Dodiya HB, Forsyth CB, Voigt RM, et al. Chronic stress-induced gut dysfunction exacerbates Parkinson's disease phenotype and pathology in a rotenone-induced mouse model of Parkinson's disease. *Neurobiol Dis.* 2020;135:104352.

6. Kelly RR, McDonald LT, Jensen NR, Sidles SJ, LaRue AC. Impacts of Psychological Stress on Osteoporosis: Clinical Implications and Treatment Interactions. *Front Psychiatry.* 2019;10:200.

7. Dennison E, Hindmarsh P, Fall C, et al. Profiles of Endogenous Circulating Cortisol and Bone Mineral Density in Healthy Elderly Men. *J Clin Endocrinol Metab.* 1999;84(9):3058-3063.

8. Reynolds RM, Dennison EM, Walker BR, et al. Cortisol secretion and rate of bone loss in a population-based cohort of elderly men and women. *Calcif Tissue Int.* 2005;77(3):134-138.

9. Burla F, Dussi S, Martinez-Torres C, Tauber J, van der Gucht J, Koenderink GH. Connectivity and plasticity determine collagen network fracture. *Proc Natl Acad Sci U S A.* 2020;117(15):8326-8334.

10. Lodish H, Berk A, Zipursky S. Section 22.3, Collagen: The Fibrous Proteins of the Matrix. In: *Molecular Cell Biology. 4th edition.* New York: W. H. Freeman; 2000.

11. Moskowitz RW. Role of collagen hydrolysate in bone and joint disease. *Semin Arthritis Rheum.* 2000;30(2):87-99.

12. Golovatscka V, Ennes H, Mayer EA, Bradesi S. Chronic stress-induced changes in pro-inflammatory cytokines and spinal glia markers in the rat: a time course study. *Neuroimmunomodulation.* 2012;19(6):367-376.

13. Cui SJ, Fu Y, Liu Y, et al. Chronic inflammation deteriorates structure and function of collagen fibril in rat temporomandibular joint disc. *Int J Oral Sci.* 2019;11(1):2.

14. Siwik DA, Chang DL, Colucci WS. Interleukin-1beta and tumor necrosis factor-alpha decrease collagen synthesis and increase matrix metalloproteinase activity in cardiac fibroblasts in vitro. *Circ Res.* 2000;86(12):1259-1265.

15. Viguet-Carrin S, Garnero P, Delmas PD. The role of collagen in bone strength. *Osteoporos Int.* 2006;17(3):319-336.

16. Wang X, Shen X, Li X, Agrawal CM. Age-related changes in the collagen network and toughness of bone. *Bone.* 2002;31(1):1-7.

17. Hansen MM, Jones R, Tocchini K. Shinrin-Yoku (Forest Bathing) and Nature Therapy: A State-of-the-Art Review. *Int J Environ Res Public Health.* 2017;14(8).

## Chapter 10

1. Sleep Disorders and Sleep Deprivation: An Unmet Public Health Problem. In: Colton H, Altevogt B, eds.: The National Academies Press; 2006:424.

2. Watson NF, Badr MS, Belenky G, et al. Joint Consensus Statement of the American Academy of Sleep Medicine and Sleep Research Society on the Recommended Amount of Sleep for a Healthy Adult: Methodology and Discussion. *Sleep.* 2015;38(8):1161-1183.

3. Banks S, Dinges DF. Behavioral and physiological consequences of sleep restriction. *J Clin Sleep Med.* 2007;3(5):519-528.

4. Ford ES, Cunningham TJ, Croft JB. Trends in Self-Reported Sleep Duration among US Adults from 1985 to 2012. *Sleep.* 2015;38(5):829-832.

5. Doghramji PP. Detection of insomnia in primary care. *The Journal of clinical psychiatry.* 2001;62 Suppl 10:18-26.

6. Hardeland R. Melatonin in aging and disease -multiple consequences of reduced secretion, options and limits of treatment. *Aging Dis.* 2012;3(2):194-225.

7. Troxel WM. It's more than sex: exploring the dyadic nature of sleep and implications for health. *Psychosom Med.* 2010;72(6):578-586.

8. Ochs-Balcom HM, Hovey KM, Andrews C, et al. Short Sleep Is Associated With Low Bone Mineral Density and Osteoporosis in the Women's Health Initiative. *J Bone Miner Res.* 2020;35(2):261-268.

9. Glass J, Lanctot KL, Herrmann N, Sproule BA, Busto UE. Sedative hypnotics in older people with insomnia: meta-analysis of risks and benefits. *BMJ.* 2005;331(7526):1169.

10. Kripke DF, Langer RD, Kline LE. Hypnotics' association with mortality or cancer: a matched cohort study. *BMJ Open.* 2012;2(1):e000850.

11. Kripke DF. Hypnotic drug risks of mortality, infection, depression, and cancer: but lack of benefit. *F1000Res.* 2016;5:918.

12. Gauld AR. Suvorexant (Belsomra) for Insomnia. *Am Fam Physician.* 2016;93(12):1016-1020.

13. Chang AM, Aeschbach D, Duffy JF, Czeisler CA. Evening use of light-emitting eReaders negatively affects sleep, circadian timing, and next-morning alertness. *Proc Natl Acad Sci U S A.* 2015;112(4):1232-1237.

14. Koseck D. How Much Sleep Do Fitbit Users Really Get? A New Study Finds Out. Fitbit News Web site. https://blog.fitbit.com/sleep-study/. Published 2017. Accessed April 30, 2018.

15. Pogue D. Exclusive: What Fitbit's 6 billion nights of sleep data reveals about us. . Yahoo Finance Web site. https://finance.yahoo.com/news/exclusive-fitbits-6-billion-nights-sleep-data-reveals-us-110058417.html. Published 2018. Accessed April 30, 2018.

16. Cheung KS, Chan EW, Wong AYS, Chen L, Wong ICK, Leung WK. Long-term proton pump inhibitors and risk of gastric cancer development after treatment for Helicobacter pylori: a population-based study. *Gut.* 2018;67(1):28-35.

17. Gomm W, von Holt K, Thomé F, et al. Association of proton pump inhibitors with risk of dementia: A pharmacoepidemiological claims data analysis. *JAMA Neurology.* 2016;73(4):410-416.

18. Yang YX, Lewis JD, Epstein S, Metz DC. Long-term proton pump inhibitor therapy and risk of hip fracture. *JAMA.* 2006;296(24):2947-2953.

19. Reid KJ, Baron KG, Lu B, Naylor E, Wolfe L, Zee PC. Aerobic exercise improves self-reported sleep and quality of life in older adults with insomnia. *Sleep Med.* 2010;11(9):934-940.

20. Medications that can affect sleep. Harvard Health Publishing. Harvard Women's Health Watch Web site. https://www.health.harvard.edu/newsletter_article/medications-that-can-affect-sleep. Published 2010. Accessed December 28, 2017.

21. Arendt J, Bojkowski C, Franey C, Wright J, Marks V. Immunoassay of 6-hydroxymelatonin sulfate in human plasma and urine: abolition of the urinary 24-hour rhythm with atenolol. *J Clin Endocrinol Metab.* 1985;60(6):1166-1173.

22. Scheer FA, Morris CJ, Garcia JI, et al. Repeated melatonin supplementation improves sleep in hypertensive patients treated with beta-blockers: a randomized controlled trial. *Sleep.* 2012;35(10):1395-1402.

## Chapter 11

1. Bolland MJ, Leung W, Tai V, et al. Calcium intake and risk of fracture: systematic review. *BMJ.* Sep 29 2015;351:h4580.

2. Larsen ER, Mosekilde L, Foldspang A. Vitamin D and Calcium Supplementation Prevents Osteoporotic Fractures in Elderly Community Dwelling Residents: A Pragmatic Population-Based 3-Year Intervention Study. *Journal of Bone and Mineral Research.* 2004;19(3):370-378.

3. Nicar MJ, Pak CY. Calcium bioavailability from calcium carbonate and calcium citrate. *J Clin Endocrinol Metab*. Aug 1985;61(2):391-3.

4. Hurwitz A, Ruhl C. Gastric Hypochlorhydria and Achlorhydria in Older Adults-Reply. *JAMA*. 1997;278(20):1659-1660.

5. van der Velde RY, Brouwers JR, Geusens PP, Lems WF, van den Bergh JP. Calcium and vitamin D supplementation: state of the art for daily practice. *Food Nutr Res*. 2014;58doi:10.3402/fnr.v58.21796.

6. Frassetto L, Kohlstadt I. Treatment and prevention of kidney stones: an update. *Am Fam Physician*. Dec 1 2011;84(11):1234-42.

7. Kopecky SL, Bauer DC, Gulati M, et al. Lack of Evidence Linking Calcium With or Without Vitamin D Supplementation to Cardiovascular Disease in Generally Healthy Adults: A Clinical Guideline From the National Osteoporosis Foundation and the American Society for Preventive Cardiology. *Ann Intern Med*. Dec 20 2016;165(12):867-868.

8. What We Eat in America. 2017-2018. U.S. Department of Agriculture, Agricultural Research Service. Accessed May 16, 2022.

9. Naeem Z. Vitamin d deficiency- an ignored epidemic. *Int J Health Sci (Qassim)*. Jan 2010;4(1):V-VI.

10. Vieth R. Vitamin D supplementation: cholecalciferol, calcifediol, and calcitriol. *European Journal of Clinical Nutrition*. 2020/11/01 2020;74(11):1493-1497.

11. Wilson LR, Tripkovic L, Hart KH, Lanham-New SA. Vitamin D deficiency as a public health issue: using vitamin D2 or vitamin D3 in future fortification strategies. *Proc Nutr Soc*. Aug 2017;76(3):392-399.

12. Holick MF. The vitamin D deficiency pandemic: Approaches for diagnosis, treatment and prevention. *Rev Endocr Metab Disord*. Jun 2017;18(2):153-165.

13. Parva NR, Tadepalli S, Singh P, et al. Prevalence of Vitamin D Deficiency and Associated Risk Factors in the US Population (2011-2012). *Cureus*. Jun 5 2018;10(6):e2741.

14. Kumar J, Muntner P, Kaskel FJ, Hailpern SM, Melamed ML. Prevalence and associations of 25-hydroxyvitamin D deficiency in US children: NHANES 2001-2004. *Pediatrics.* Sep 2009;124(3):e362-70.

15. Time for more vitamin D. Web page. Harvard Health Publishing. Accessed February 26, 2022.

16. Holick MF. Vitamin D: importance in the prevention of cancers, type 1 diabetes, heart disease, and osteoporosis. *Am J Clin Nutr.* Mar 2004;79(3):362-71.

17. Holick MF. Vitamin D deficiency. *N Engl J Med.* Jul 19 2007;357(3):266-81.

18. Melamed ML, Michos ED, Post W, Astor B. 25-hydroxyvitamin D levels and the risk of mortality in the general population. *Arch Intern Med.* Aug 11 2008;168(15):1629-37.

19. Bjelakovic G, Gluud LL, Nikolova D, et al. Vitamin D supplementation for prevention of mortality in adults. *Cochrane Database Syst Rev.* Jan 10 2014;(1):Cd007470.

20. Cranney A, Horsley T, O'Donnell S, et al. Effectiveness and safety of vitamin D in relation to bone health. *Evid Rep Technol Assess (Full Rep).* Aug 2007;(158):1-235.

21. Bischoff-Ferrari HA, Shao A, Dawson-Hughes B, Hathcock J, Giovannucci E, Willett WC. Benefit-risk assessment of vitamin D supplementation. *Osteoporos Int.* Jul 2010;21(7):1121-32.

22. McDonnell SL, Baggerly CA, French CB, et al. Breast cancer risk markedly lower with serum 25-hydroxyvitamin D concentrations ≥60 vs <20 ng/ml (150 vs 50 nmol/L): Pooled analysis of two randomized trials and a prospective cohort. *PloS one.* 2018;13(6):e0199265-e0199265.

23. Holick MF, Biancuzzo RM, Chen TC, et al. Vitamin D2 is as effective as vitamin D3 in maintaining circulating concentrations of 25-hydroxyvitamin D. *J Clin Endocrinol Metab.* Mar 2008;93(3):677-81.

24. Heaney RP, Davies KM, Chen TC, Holick MF, Barger-Lux MJ. Human serum 25-hydroxycholecalciferol response to extended oral dosing with cholecalciferol. *Am J Clin Nutr.* Jan 2003;77(1):204-10.

25. Heaney RP, Davies KM, Chen TC, Holick MF, Barger-Lux MJ. Human serum 25-hydroxycholecalciferol response to extended oral dosing with cholecalciferol. *The American Journal of Clinical Nutrition.* 2003;77(1):204-210.

26. Bischoff-Ferrari HA. The 25-hydroxyvitamin D threshold for better health. *The Journal of Steroid Biochemistry and Molecular Biology.* 2007;103(3-5):614-619.

27. Hathcock JN, Shao A, Vieth R, Heaney R. Risk assessment for vitamin D. *Am J Clin Nutr.* Jan 2007;85(1):6-18.

28. Ross AC, Taylor CL, Yaktine AL, Del Valle HB, eds. *Dietary Reference Intakes for Calcium and Vitamin D.* National Academies Press (US); 2011.

29. Vitamin D: Fact Sheet for Health Professionals. National Insitutes of Health Office of Dietary Supplements. Accessed May 12, 2022.

30. Weydert JA. Vitamin D in Children's Health. *Children.* 2014;1(2):208-226.

31. Marcinowska-Suchowierska E, Kupisz-Urbańska M, Łukaszkiewicz J, Płudowski P, Jones G. Vitamin D Toxicity—A Clinical Perspective. Review. *Frontiers in Endocrinology.* 2018-September-20 2018;9

32. Shearer MJ, Newman P. Metabolism and cell biology of vitamin K. *Thromb Haemost.* 2008;100(4):530-47.

33. Shearer MJ, Newman P. Recent trends in the metabolism and cell biology of vitamin K with special reference to vitamin K cycling and MK-4 biosynthesis. *J Lipid Res.* Mar 2014;55(3):345-62.

34. Ronden JE, Drittij-Reijnders M-J, Vermeer C, Thijssen HHW. Intestinal flora is not an intermediate in the phylloquinone-menaquinone-4 conversion in the rat. *Biochimica et Biophysica Acta (BBA) - General Subjects.* 1998;1379(1):69-75.

35. Davidson RT, Foley AL, Engelke JA, Suttie JW. Conversion of Dietary Phylloquinone to Tissue Menaquinone-4 in Rats is Not Dependent on Gut Bacteria1. *J Nutr.* 1998;128(2):220-223.

36. Iwamoto I, Kosha S, Noguchi S-i. A longitudinal study of the effect of vitamin K2 on bone mineral density in postmenopausal women a comparative study with vitamin D3 and estrogen-progestin therapy. *Maturitas*. 1999;31(2):161-164.

37. Shiraki M, Shiraki Y, Aoki C, Miura M. Vitamin K2 (Menatetrenone) Effectively Prevents Fractures and Sustains Lumbar Bone Mineral Density in Osteoporosis. *Journal of Bone and Mineral Research*. 2000;15(3):515-522.

38. Cockayne S, Adamson J, Lanham-New S, Shearer MJ, Gilbody S, Torgerson DJ. Vitamin K and the Prevention of Fractures: Systematic Review and Meta-analysis of Randomized Controlled Trials. *Arch Intern Med*. 2006;166(12):1256-1261.

39. Huang ZB, Wan SL, Lu YJ, Ning L, Liu C, Fan SW. Does vitamin K2 play a role in the prevention and treatment of osteoporosis for postmenopausal women: a meta-analysis of randomized controlled trials. *Osteoporosis International*. 2015/03/01 2015;26(3):1175-1186.

40. Ushiroyama T, Ikeda A, Ueki M. Effect of continuous combined therapy with vitamin K2 and vitamin D3 on bone mineral density and coagulofibrinolysis function in postmenopausal women. *Maturitas*. 2002;41(3):211-221.

41. Purwosunu Y, Muharram, Rachman IA, Reksoprodjo S, Sekizawa A. Vitamin K2 treatment for postmenopausal osteoporosis in Indonesia. *J Obstet Gynaecol Res*. Apr 2006;32(2):230-4.

42. Iwamoto J, Takeda T, Ichimura S. Effect of combined administration of vitamin D3 and vitamin K2 on bone mineral density of the lumbar spine in postmenopausal women with osteoporosis. *J Orthop Sci*. 2000;5(6):546-51.

43. Sasaki N, Kusano E, Takahashi H, et al. Vitamin K2 inhibits glucocorticoid-induced bone loss partly by preventing the reduction of osteoprotegerin (OPG). *Journal of bone and mineral metabolism*. 2005;23(1):41-7.

44. Yonemura K, Fukasawa H, Fujigaki Y, Hishida A. Protective effect of vitamins K2 and D3 on prednisolone-induced loss of bone mineral density in the lumbar spine. *Am J Kidney Dis*. Jan 2004;43(1):53-60.

45. Yonemura K, Kimura M, Miyaji T, Hishida A. Short-term effect of vitamin K administration on prednisolone-induced loss of bone mineral density in patients with chronic glomerulonephritis. *Calcified tissue international*. Feb 2000;66(2):123-8.

46. Inoue T, Sugiyama T, Matsubara T, Kawai S, Furukawa S. Inverse correlation between the changes of lumbar bone mineral density and serum undercarboxylated osteocalcin after vitamin K2 (menatetrenone) treatment in children treated with glucocorticoid and alfacalcidol. *Endocrine journal*. Feb 2001;48(1):11-8.

47. Iketani T, Kiriike N, Murray, et al. Effect of menatetrenone (vitamin K2) treatment on bone loss in patients with anorexia nervosa. *Psychiatry Res*. Mar 25 2003;117(3):259-69.

48. Shiomi S, Nishiguchi S, Kubo S. Vitamin K2 (menatetrenone) for bone loss in patients with cirrhosis of the liver. *The American Journal of Gastroenterology*. 2002;97(4):978-981.

49. Sato Y, Honda Y, Kuno H, Oizumi K. Menatetrenone ameliorates osteopenia in disuse-affected limbs of vitamin D- and K-deficient stroke patients. *Bone*. Sep 1998;23(3):291-6.

50. Nishiguchi S, Shimoi S, Kurooka H. Randomized pilot trial of vitamin K2 for bone loss in patients with primary biliary cirrhosis. *Journal of Hepatology*. 2001;35(4):543-545.

51. Somekawa Y, Chigughi M, Harada M, Ishibashi T. Use of vitamin K2 (menatetrenone) and 1,25-dihydroxyvitamin D3 in the prevention of bone loss induced by leuprolide. *J Clin Endocrinol Metab*. Aug 1999;84(8):2700-4.

52. Fujishiro A, Iwasa M, Fujii S, et al. Menatetrenone facilitates hematopoietic cell generation in a manner that is dependent on human bone marrow mesenchymal stromal/stem cells. *Int J Hematol*. Sep 2020;112(3):316-330.

53. Carrié I, Portoukalian J, Vicaretti R, Rochford J, Potvin S, Ferland G. Menaquinone-4 Concentration Is Correlated with Sphingolipid Concentrations in Rat Brain. *The Journal of Nutrition*. 2004;134(1):167-172.

54. Ferland G. Vitamin K and brain function. *Semin Thromb Hemost.* Nov 2013;39(8):849-55.

55. Ide Y, Zhang H, Hamajima H, et al. Inhibition of matrix metalloproteinase expression by menatetrenone, a vitamin K2 analogue. *Oncol Rep.* 2009;22(3):599-604.

56. Ozaki I, Zhang H, Mizuta T, et al. Menatetrenone, a Vitamin K2 Analogue, Inhibits Hepatocellular Carcinoma Cell Growth by Suppressing Cyclin D1 Expression through Inhibition of Nuclear Factor kB Activation. *Clinical Cancer Research.* 2007;13(7):2236-2245.

57. Naim A, Pan Q, Baig MS. Matrix Metalloproteinases (MMPs) in Liver Diseases. *J Clin Exp Hepatol.* 2017;7(4):367-372.

58. Asakura H, Myou S, Ontachi Y. Vitamin K administration to elderly patients with osteoporosis induces no hemostatic activation, even in those with suspected vitamin K deficiency. *Osteoporos Int.* Dec 2001;12(12):996-1000.

59. Buehler MJ. Nature designs tough collagen: Explaining the nanostructure of collagen fibrils. *Proceedings of the National Academy of Sciences.* 2006;103(33):12285-12290.

60. Tzaphlidou M. Bone architecture: collagen structure and calcium/phosphorus maps. *J Biol Phys.* 2008;34(1-2):39-49.

61. Authority EFS. Opinion of the Scientific Panel on biological hazards (BIOHAZ) on the safety of collagen and a processing method for the production of collagen. *EFSA Journal.* 2005;3(3):174.

62. Guillerminet F, Beaupied H, Fabien-Soulé V, et al. Hydrolyzed collagen improves bone metabolism and biomechanical parameters in ovariectomized mice: an in vitro and in vivo study. *Bone.* Mar 2010;46(3):827-34.

63. Figueres Juher T, Basés Pérez E. [An overview of the beneficial effects of hydrolysed collagen intake on joint and bone health and on skin ageing]. *Nutr Hosp.* Jul 18 2015;32 Suppl 1:62-6.

64. Tsuruoka N, Yamato R, Sakai Y, Yoshitake Y, Yonekura H. Promotion by collagen tripeptide of type I collagen gene expression in human osteoblastic cells and fracture healing of rat femur. *Biosci Biotechnol Biochem.* Nov 2007;71(11):2680-7.

65. Vasikaran S, Eastell R, Bruyère O, et al. Markers of bone turnover for the prediction of fracture risk and monitoring of osteoporosis treatment: a need for international reference standards. *Osteoporos Int.* Feb 2011;22(2):391-420.

66. Garnero P, Sornay-Rendu E, Claustrat B, Delmas PD. Biochemical markers of bone turnover, endogenous hormones and the risk of fractures in postmenopausal women: the OFELY study. *J Bone Miner Res.* Aug 2000;15(8):1526-36.

67. Chapurlat RD, Garnero P, Bréart G, Meunier PJ, Delmas PD. Serum type I collagen breakdown product (serum CTX) predicts hip fracture risk in elderly women: the EPIDOS study. *Bone.* Aug 2000;27(2):283-6.

68. Argyrou C, Karlafti E, Lampropoulou-Adamidou K, et al. Effect of calcium and vitamin D supplementation with and without collagen peptides on bone turnover in postmenopausal women with osteopenia. *Journal of musculoskeletal & neuronal interactions.* 2020;20(1):12-17.

69. Li T, Jiang S, Lu C, et al. Melatonin: Another avenue for treating osteoporosis? *J Pineal Res.* Mar 2019;66(2):e12548.

70. Amstrup AK, Sikjaer T, Heickendorff L, Mosekilde L, Rejnmark L. Melatonin improves bone mineral density at the femoral neck in postmenopausal women with osteopenia: a randomized controlled trial. *J Pineal Res.* Sep 2015;59(2):221-9.

71. Marie PJ, Hott M, Modrowski D, et al. An uncoupling agent containing strontium prevents bone loss by depressing bone resorption and maintaining bone formation in estrogen-deficient rats. *J Bone Miner Res.* May 1993;8(5):607-15.

72. Caverzasio J. Strontium ranelate promotes osteoblastic cell replication through at least two different mechanisms. *Bone.* 2008;42(6):1131-1136.

73. Meunier PJ, Slosman DO, Delmas PD, et al. Strontium ranelate: dose-dependent effects in established postmenopausal vertebral osteoporosis--a 2-year randomized placebo controlled trial. *J Clin Endocrinol Metab.* 2002;87(5):2060-6.

74. Meunier PJ, Roux C, Seeman E, et al. The Effects of Strontium Ranelate on the Risk of Vertebral Fracture in Women with Postmenopausal Osteoporosis. *N Engl J Med*. 2004;350(5):459-468.

75. Moise H, Chettle DR, Pejović-Milić A. Monitoring bone strontium intake in osteoporotic females self-supplementing with strontium citrate with a novel in-vivo X-ray fluorescence based diagnostic tool. *Bone*. Apr 2014;61:48-54.

76. Bolland MJ, Grey A. A comparison of adverse event and fracture efficacy data for strontium ranelate in regulatory documents and the publication record. *BMJ Open*. Oct 7 2014;4(10):e005787.

77. Stendig-Lindberg G, Tepper R, Leichter I. Trabecular bone density in a two year controlled trial of peroral magnesium in osteoporosis. *Magnes Res*. Jun 1993;6(2):155-63.

78. Orchard TS, Larson JC, Alghothani N, et al. Magnesium intake, bone mineral density, and fractures: results from the Women's Health Initiative Observational Study. *Am J Clin Nutr*. Apr 2014;99(4):926-33.

79. Ames BN. Low micronutrient intake may accelerate the degenerative diseases of aging through allocation of scarce micronutrients by triage. *PNAS*. 2006;103(47):17589-17594.

80. Siscovick DS, Barringer TA, Fretts AM, et al. Omega-3 Polyunsaturated Fatty Acid (Fish Oil) Supplementation and the Prevention of Clinical Cardiovascular Disease. *Circulation*. 2017;135(15):e867-e884.

81. Shahidi F, Ambigaipalan P. Omega-3 Polyunsaturated Fatty Acids and Their Health Benefits. *Annu Rev Food Sci Technol*. Mar 25 2018;9:345-381.

## Chapter 12

1. Lee S, Seo DH, Kim KM, et al. Contingent association between the size of the social support network and osteoporosis among Korean elderly women. *PLoS One*. 2017;12(7):e0180017.

2. Mezuk B, Eaton WW, Golden SH. Depression and osteoporosis: epidemiology and potential mediating pathways. *Osteoporos Int*. 2008;19(1):1-12.

3. Michelson D, Stratakis C, Hill L, et al. Bone mineral density in women with depression. *N Engl J Med.* 1996;335(16):1176-1181.

4. Ganesan K, Teklehaimanot S, Tran TH, Asuncion M, Norris K. Relationship of C-reactive protein and bone mineral density in community-dwelling elderly females. *J Natl Med Assoc.* 2005;97(3):329-333.

5. Resnick B, Orwig D, Magaziner J, Wynne C. The effect of social support on exercise behavior in older adults. *Clin Nurs Res.* 2002;11(1):52-70.

6. Kaplan RM, Hartwell SL. Differential effects of social support and social network on physiological and social outcomes in men and women with type II diabetes mellitus. *Health Psychol.* 1987;6(5):387-398.

7. Tan J, Wang Y. Social Integration, Social Support, and All-Cause, Cardiovascular Disease and Cause-Specific Mortality: A Prospective Cohort Study. *Int J Environ Res Public Health.* 2019;16(9).

8. Follis SL, Bea J, Klimentidis Y, et al. Psychosocial stress and bone loss among postmenopausal women: results from the Women's Health Initiative. *J Epidemiol Community Health.* 2019;73(9):888-892.

9. Ma L, Li Y, Wang J, et al. Quality of Life Is Related to Social Support in Elderly Osteoporosis Patients in a Chinese Population. *PLoS One.* 2015;10(6):e0127849.

10. Perissinotto CM, Stijacic Cenzer I, Covinsky KE. Loneliness in older persons: a predictor of functional decline and death. *Arch Intern Med.* 2012;172(14):1078-1083.

11. McGinty EE, Presskreischer R, Han H, Barry CL. Psychological Distress and Loneliness Reported by US Adults in 2018 and April 2020. *Jama.* 2020;324(1):93-94.

12. Burr JA, Han SH, Tavares JL. Volunteering and Cardiovascular Disease Risk: Does Helping Others Get "Under the Skin?". *The Gerontologist.* 2016;56(5):937-947.

13. Thoits PA, Hewitt LN. Volunteer work and well-being. *J Health Soc Behav.* 2001;42(2):115-131.

14. Konrath S, Fuhrel-Forbis A, Lou A, Brown S. Motives for volunteering are associated with mortality risk in older adults. *Health Psychol.* 2012;31(1):87-96.

15. Yeung JWK, Zhang Z, Kim TY. Volunteering and health benefits in general adults: cumulative effects and forms. *BMC Public Health.* 2017;18(1):8.

16. Wang Y, Ge J, Zhang H, Wang H, Xie X. Altruistic behaviors relieve physical pain. *Proceedings of the National Academy of Sciences.* 2020;117(2):950-958.

17. Harbaugh WT, Mayr U, Burghart DR. Neural responses to taxation and voluntary giving reveal motives for charitable donations. *Science.* 2007;316(5831):1622-1625.

18. Salt E, Crofford LJ, Segerstrom S. The Mediating and Moderating Effect of Volunteering on Pain and Depression, Life Purpose, Well-Being, and Physical Activity. *Pain Management Nursing.* 2017;18(4):243-249.

Use these tables to understand if you're eating enough plants and protein. You can download PDFs of the tables at nbi-health.com/osteobook.

## Plants

Plants contain fiber that helps regulate your blood sugar, promotes healthy gut bacteria, helps you feel full longer and bulks up your stools for healthy poop. The two main types of fiber are soluble and insoluble fiber. To get a healthy mix of fibers and other important plant nutrients, eat a rainbow a day of richly colored fruits, vegetable, grains and legumes.

The goal is to eat at least 30 grams of total dietary fiber a day. Here are some tips:

- Include fruits and vegetables in your diet. Increase vegetable consumption to at least three servings per day. Increase fruit consumption to at least two servings per day.
- Snack on fresh fruits and vegetables in place of sugary or refined foods.
- Increase whole grain consumption to at least four servings per day. Include oats, brown rice, bran, quinoa, barley and whole wheat. Choose whole grains and avoid white flour products.

- Add oat bran, wheat germ or rice bran to hot cereal or yogurt.
- Add bran cereal or oatmeal to meat loaf, meatballs or hamburgers.
- Eat legumes daily. Replace creamy dips and spreads with bean dips or spreads such as hummus, black bean dip or refried beans.

Since increasing your fiber too quickly can create gas and bloating, work up to the recommended amount over a week or two. Making sure you're drinking plenty of water—at least 8 glasses per day—can help you avoid the discomfort that can occur with a sudden increase in fiber.

| Fruits | Serving Size | Total Fiber (grams)* |
|---|---|---|
| Apple, with skin | 1 medium | 4.1 |
| Banana | 1 medium | 3.1 |
| Pear, with skin | 1 medium | 5.5 |
| Orange | 1 large | 4.4 |
| Prunes, pitted and dried | 1 cup | 12.4 |
| Strawberries, halved | 1 cup | 3.0 |
| **Vegetables** | | |
| Broccoli, cooked | 1 cup | 5.5 |
| Carrots | 1 large | 2.0 |
| Corn, yellow | 1 cup | 12.0 |
| Kale, cooked | 1 cup | 2.7 |
| Potato, baked with skin | 1 medium | 4.0 |
| Spinach, cooked | 1 cup | 5.5 |
| Swiss chard | 1 cup | 0.6 |

| Beans, legumes, nuts and seeds | Serving Size | Total Fiber (grams)* |
|---|---|---|
| Black beans, cooked | 1 cup | 11 |
| Garbanzo beans, cooked | 1 cup | 12 |
| Green peas, cooked | 2/3 cup | 3.9 |
| Kidney beans, cooked | 1 cup | 13 |
| Lentils, cooked | 2/3 cup | 4.5 |
| Lima beans, cooked | 1 cup | 13 |
| Pinto beans, cooked | 1 cup | 14 |
| Peanut butter, chunky | 2 tbsp | 1.5 |
| Psyllium seeds, ground | 1 tbsp | 6.0 |
| Refried beans, Amy's® vegetarian | 1/2 cup | 6.0 |
| **Nuts & Seeds** | | |
| Almonds | 1 cup | 18 |
| Almond butter | 2 Tbsp | 3.3 |
| Cashews | 1 cup | 4.0 |
| Peanut butter, chunky | 2 Tbsp | 2.5 |
| Peanut butter, smooth | 2 Tbsp | 1.6 |
| Peanuts | 1 oz | 2.4 |
| Pumpkin seeds | 1 cup | 12 |
| Sunflower seeds | 1 oz | 3.3 |
| **Whole grains** | | |
| Bagel, Plain (Dave's Killer Bread®) | 1 bagel | 11 |
| Barley, cooked | 1 cup | 6.0 |
| Bread, flourless sprouted grain (Ezekiel 4:9®) | 1 slice | 3.0 |
| Brown rice, uncooked | 1 cup | 6.6 |
| Cereal, Sprouted Flourless Flake (Ezekiel 4:9®) | ¾ cup | 6.0 |
| Mary's Gone Crackers® Original | 12 crackers | 3.0 |
| Oats, cooked rolled oats | ¾ cup | 3.0 |
| White rice, uncooked | 1 cup | 2.4 |

*Sources: US Department of Agriculture FoodData Central (https://fdc.nal.usda.gov/index.html) and Nutrition Facts panels for packaged foods.

## Protein

To build stronger bones and muscles, the research suggests a minimum protein intake of 1.3 grams per kilogram (g/kg) body weight per day, plus resistance training. Other recommendations go as high as 2.0 g/kg body weight per day.

In Chapter 7 you calculated the number of grams of protein you should be eating per day. Write it down here:

**_____ grams of protein per day.**

| Beans/Legumes – 1 cup cooked | | | |
|---|---|---|---|
| Adzuki beans | 17 g | Lentils | 16 g |
| Black beans | 15 g | Pinto beans | 14 g |
| Black-eyed peas | 13 g | Refried beans, Amy's® | 8 g |
| Garbanzo beans | 14 g | vegetarian | |
| Kidney beans | 18 g | Split peas | 16 g |
| **Dairy, Soy & Substitute Products** | | | |
| Cottage cheese, 1 cup | 31 g | Milk, 2%, 1 cup | 8 g |
| Tofu, firm, 4 oz | 20 g | Cheese, 1 oz | 7 g |
| Tempeh, 3 oz | 16 g | Soy cheese, 1 oz | 6 g |
| Yogurt, low fat, 1 cup | 10 g | Soy burger, 1 patty, 4 oz | 14 g |
| Yogurt, whole milk plain | 16 g | Miso paste, 2 Tbsp | 4 g |
| Greek yogurt, 1 cup | | Cream cheese, 1 oz | 3 g |
| Soy yogurt, 1 cup | 9 g | Soy milk, 1 cup | 6 g |
| Goat milk, 1 cup | 9 g | Rice milk, 1 cup | 1 g |
| Milk, skim, 1 cup | 8 g | | |

| Grains (1 cup cooked) & Grain Products | | | |
|---|---|---|---|
| Amaranth | 14 g | Brown rice, raw | 14 g |
| Bagel, Plain | 11 g | White rice, raw | 13 g |
| (Dave's Killer Bread®) | | Oatmeal | 5 g |
| Barley | 16 g | Quinoa | 22 g |
| Bread, flourless sprouted | 5 g | Mary's Gone Crackers® | 4 g |
| grain (Ezekiel 4:9) | | Original | |
| Cereal, Flourless Flake | 8 g | Millet | 8 g |
| (Ezekiel 4:9) | | | |
| English muffin, | 6 g | | |
| (Dave's Killer Bread) | | | |

**Meats, Seafood, & Poultry – 3 oz**
**(about the size of a deck of cards in the palm of your hand)**

| | | | |
|---|---|---|---|
| Beef, lean | 22 g | Ham | 18 g |
| Chicken Breast | 26 g | Hamburger | 21 g |
| Clams | 22 g | Pork chop | 19 g |
| Crabmeat | 16 g | Salmon | 20 g |
| Egg, 1 | 7 g | Tuna, in water | 22 g |
| Fish, white | 17 g | Turkey | 25 g |

| Nuts & Seeds | | | |
|---|---|---|---|
| Almonds, 1 cup | 30 g | Peanut butter, smooth, 2 | 7 g |
| Almond butter, 2 Tbsp | 7 g | Tbsp | 7 g |
| Cashews, 1 cup | 21 g | Peanuts, 1 oz | 12 g |
| Peanut butter, chunky, 2 | 8 g | Pumpkin seeds, 1 cup | 5 g |
| Tbsp | | Sunflower seeds, 1 oz | |

# Appendix B: Calcium Content of Foods

The US Recommended Daily Amount (RDA) of calcium for women is 1,000 mg per day until they reach 50 years old, then increases to 1,200 mg. For men up to 70 years old, it's 1,000 mg per day, then 1,200 mg after that.

| Fruits and Vegetables (1 cup, unless otherwise stated) | | | |
|---|---|---|---|
| Avocado, 1 medium | 30 mg | Mustard greens, cooked | 450 mg |
| Bean sprouts | 320 mg | Okra, sliced, boiled | 100 mg |
| Beans, green, snap, boiled | 58 mg | Onions, chopped, raw | 32 mg |
| Beans, wax, cut, canned | 174 mg | Parsley, chopped, raw | 82 mg |
| Beet greens, boiled | 165 mg | Parsley, sliced, boiled | 912 mg |
| Blackberries, raw | 46 mg | Parsnips, sliced, boiled | 58 mg |
| Blueberries, frozen, unsweetened | 44 mg | Peas, green, raw | 36 mg |
| Bok choy, cooked | 330 mg | Potato, w/skin baked, 1 medium | 20 mg |
| Bok choy, raw | 250 mg | Pumpkin, canned | 64 mg |
| Borage, boiled | 235 mg | Rhubarb, frozen, raw | 266 mg |
| Broccoli, raw | 160 mg | Rutabaga, cubed, boiled | 72 mg |
| Brussel sprouts, boiled | 56 mg | Salsify, sliced, boiled | 64 mg |
| Cabbage, shredded, raw | 32 mg | Sauerkraut, canned | 72 mg |
| Carrots , sliced, boiled | 48 mg | Shallots, chopped, raw | 64 mg |
| Cassava, raw | 209 mg | Shepherds Purse, cooked | 300 mg |
| Cauliflower, pieces, raw | 28 mg | Snow peas, raw | 62 mg |
| Celeriac, raw | 99 mg | Spinach, chopped, raw | 80 mg |
| Celery, diced, boiled | 64 mg | Spinach, cooked | 250 mg |
| Collard greens, cooked | 360 mg | Squash | |
| Dandelion greens, boiled | 146 mg | Acorn squash, cubed, baked | 90 mg |
| Eggplant, raw | 30 mg | Butternut squash, boiled | 84 mg |

| | | | |
|---|---|---|---|
| Fennel bulb, sliced, raw | 43 mg | Hubbard/Spaghetti squash | 34 mg |
| Garden cress, raw | 40 mg | Sweet potato, baked w/ skin, 1 medium | 32 mg |
| Kale, fresh, chopped, steamed | 210 mg | Swiss chard | 125 mg |
| Kohlrabi, sliced, boiled | 76 mg | Turnip, cubed, boiled | 36 mg |
| Lambsquarters, chopped, steamed | 464 mg | Turnip greens, cooked | 450 mg |
| Leeks, chopped, raw | 60 mg | Watercress, chopped, raw | 40 mg |

**Beans, dried & boiled (1 cup, unless otherwise stated)**

| | | | |
|---|---|---|---|
| Adzuki beans | 63 mg | Mung beans | 55 mg |
| Black Bean | 47 mg | Navy beans | 128 mg |
| Broadbeans (fava) | 62 mg | Pinto beans | 95 mg |
| Chickpeas/Garbanzos | 340 mg | Refried beans, canned | 118 mg |
| Cowpeas/blackeye peas | 212 mg | Soybeans, mature | 175 mg |
| Cranberry beans | 89 mg | Split peas | 20 mg |
| Kidney beans | 50 mg | White beans | 161 mg |
| Lentils | 70 mg | | |

**Nuts, Nut Butters, Seeds (1 cup, unless otherwise stated)**

| | | | |
|---|---|---|---|
| Almond Butters | 670 mg | Pecans | 80 mg |
| Almonds | 660 mg | Pine nuts | 56 mg |
| Brazilnuts | 400 mg | Pistachios, shelled | 304 mg |
| Butternuts | 120 mg | Pumpkin seeds, dried | 96 mg |
| Cashew butter | 96 mg | Safflower kernels, dried | 176 mg |
| Cashews | 104 mg | Sesame seeds, 1 Tbsp | 70 mg |
| Coconut milk | 36 mg | Soybean nuts, dry roasted | 426 mg |
| Filberts/Hazelnuts | 450 mg | Sunflower butter | 120 mg |
| Flax seeds, linseed | 616 mg | Sunflower seeds | 260 mg |
| Hickory nuts | 136 mg | Tahini, sesame butter | 426 mg |
| Macadamia nuts | 160 mg | Walnuts | 280 mg |

| Dairy Products (1 cup, unless otherwise stated) | | | |
|---|---|---|---|
| Goat milk | 315 mg | Ice cream | 200 mg |
| Buttermilk | 300 mg | Butter, 1 Tbsp | 45 mg |
| Whole milk | 290 mg | Swiss cheese, 1 oz | 260 mg |
| Yogurt | 270 mg | Cheddar cheese, 1 oz | 215 mg |
| Cottage cheese | 230 mg | Parmesan cheese, 1 Tbsp | 70 mg |
| **Soy Products (1 cup, unless otherwise stated)** | | | |
| Miso | 184 mg | Tofu | 260 mg |
| Tempeh | 154 mg | Tofu, firm | 516 mg |
| **Fish (1 cup, unless otherwise stated)** | | | |
| Raw oysters | 300 mg | Mackerel canned w/ bones | 680 mg |
| Shrimp | 130 mg | Sardines canned w/ bones | 1000 mg |
| Salmon w/ bones | 490 mg | | |
| **Sprouts (1 cup, unless otherwise stated)** | | | |
| Alfalfa | 25 mg | Mung | 35 mg |

# Acknowledgments

A book, like a healthy, fulfilled life, doesn't happen because of one person. And all the knowledge and wisdom I've tried to share didn't happen because of me. It's because of the countless gifts I've received over decades from many people who have shaped how I think, what I know and who I am. If it weren't for all the people I'm about to list, this book would not have been written.

I'm forever grateful to the founders of my medical school, Bastyr University—Drs. Les Griffith, William A. Mitchell, Jr., Joseph E. Pizzorno and Sheila Quinn. Your vision of creating an accredited natural health sciences school—that's now recognized as the leading health arts and sciences university in the world—gave me a solid foundation of scientifically rigorous training and naturopathic medical philosophy. I'm forever indebted to Dr. Pizzorno, who saw my potential while in medical school, hired me as a researcher and project manager for his company and, in his role as Editor-in-Chief of Integrative Medicine: A Clinician's Journal, invited me to write medical articles for the journal. I count myself fortunate to also have had him and Dr. Mitchell as medical school professors. They poured into me and made an indelible mark on my career.

To Dr. Steven Overman, an outstanding rheumatologist and my clinical supervisor at Northwest Hospital in Seattle, Washington. You were the first conventionally trained medical doctor to show me what an integrative medicine approach to chronic diseases could look like and how MDs and NDs could share best practices and work collaboratively to improve patient care.

Thomas Dorman, MD's brilliant mind and unwavering dedication to his patients showed me the type of clinician I wanted to become. I was the first naturopathic medical student he allowed to intern in his clinic. He required I read his orthopedics textbook and watch his training videos before testing me on my knowledge of anatomy and general medicine. Only after I passed did he take me under his wing. He pushed me harder than any other supervising doc, and for that I'm eternally grateful. He was taken from this world too early. I hope he's looking down and is proud of his student.

To Dawn Sinkule, thank you for reviewing the manuscript. Your perspective helped me understand how people without medical backgrounds might receive the book and if I was communicating the information clearly enough. And thank you for leading NBI's marketing efforts, which freed up more of my time to focus on writing this book.

My business and life coach, Cathy Hanlin who helped me clarify my goals and work toward them more efficiently. You taught me how to reframe challenges into opportunities. Your system of managing my time has made me more efficient, more effective and more able to help more people with less stress.

To Penelope Wasserman, the founder of Million Dollar Bones, thank you for reviewing this manuscript. Your input and edits were invaluable. Without your insights and edits, Chapter 8 would have been missing important information.

I'm forever grateful to my patients for trusting me with their pain, struggles, hopes and intimate details of their lives. Allowing me to help you has been one of the greatest honors of my life.

To my NBI customers, thank you for letting the products I researched and formulated be part of your health routine. Your purchases not only support my work and allow me to wake up every day and do what I love, a portion goes to making integrative medicine more accessible to women, children and families.

To Lori and Steve Bush, it's difficult to sum up the importance and impact of the time we've spent together. You've both been generous with your encouragement and insights on business and human nature. You helped me understand how to lead a company with grace and humility, while also being uncompromising on product quality and the customer experience. I wouldn't have traded our meals and late-night conversations for anything.

Alison Pandev, you exemplify the philosophy of treating others how you'd like to be treated. As the customer-facing lead of NBI, you not only help people get the products and information they need to improve their health, you also freed me up so I could focus more time and energy on writing this book.

To Clint McKinlay, your belief in what I was creating with NBI and your perspective as a fellow CEO have helped keep me focused on building my business through the difficult years. Thank you for being a bright light through some dark times.

Nate and Bebe, watching you grow reminds me every day of the importance of working to leave the world a better place. This book is one of my attempts to do that, and I hope it makes you proud. Thank you both for your patience with your dad while I once again threw myself into a project. As you're starting to learn, it's so worth it. And Bebe, a special thanks for telling me to use the GoodNotes app for the book outline to organize my thoughts. You saved me countless hours of work and made my writing more efficient and enjoyable.

To the Love of My Life, Romi. Thank you for being my editor, my cheerleader and my rock. You've been my biggest fan for 21 years and believed in me when I didn't believe in myself. You inspire me to constantly strive to become a better husband, father, friend and entrepreneur. I can't imagine doing life without you.

# Want More of Dr. Neustadt?

Read his blog at nbihealth.com.

Follow him on Instagram, Facebook
and LinkedIn at @JohnNeustadt and
on TikTok at @drjohnnbi.

Listen to him read this book on Audible.

Subscribe to his newsletter at nbihealth.com.

If you enjoyed this book, please spend a few
minutes writing a review on Amazon.

# Other Books by Dr. Neustadt

*A Revolution in Health*
*through Nutritional Biochemistry*

*A Revolution in Health, Part 2:*
*How to Take Charge of Your Health*

*Foundations and Applications of Medical*
*Biochemistry in Clinical Practice*

Made in the USA
Monee, IL
25 January 2024

51909088R00131